1997

IMPROVING HEALTH CARE of the POOR

IMPROVING HEALTH CARE of the POOR

The New York City Experience

Eli Ginzberg,
Howard Berliner,
and
Miriam Ostow

Transaction Publishers
New Brunswick (U.S.A) and London (U.K.)

Library of Congress Catalog Number: 96-41534
ISBN: 1-56000-288-3
Printed in the United States of America

Library of Congress Cataloging-in-Publication Data

Ginzberg, Eli, 1911–
    Improving health care of the poor : the New York City experience / Eli Ginzberg, Howard Berliner, and Miriam Ostow.
        p. cm.
    Includes bibliographical references and index.
    ISBN 1-56000-288-3 (cloth : alk. paper)
    1. Poor—Medical care—New York (State)—New York. 2. Medical care—New York (State)—New York (State)—New York—Finance. 3. Medical care—Utilization—New York (State)—New York. 4. Medicaid—New York (State)—New York. 5. Medicare—New York (State)—New York. I. Berliner, Howard S., 1949– . II. Ostow, Miriam. III. Title.
RA398.A4N75   1996
362.1'0425—dc20   96-41534
                                                             CIP

For Daniel Patrick Moynihan
Distinguished Senior Senator from New York,
lifetime advocate for the poor,
major contributor to the realm of ideas and action

Contents

List of Tables

Preface

Exploring in late 1992-early 1993 the subject of our next inquiry into health policy with our long-term sponsor, the Robert Wood Johnson Foundation, we agreed that an in-depth examination of the health care financing and delivery system of New York City would be a useful and timely project. There were several, mutually reinforcing reasons for this choice.

President Clinton had announced his intention to make health care reform, specifically the adoption of universal health insurance, his top domestic priority. It appeared to us that a close look at New York City's long-standing commitment to provide health care to all its residents regardless of ability to pay might shed important light on the about-to-be launched national health insurance program.

Further, we knew that for the three decades following the passage of Medicare and Medicaid, increasing sums of money had become available to expand health care services to the American people. However, relatively few studies had been undertaken to assess the extent to which access to health care had improved for different groups, middle class and poor. And that appeared to be a subject worth exploring in depth. It was also in accord with the long-term research interests of the staff of the Eisenhower Center, Columbia University, that had undertaken since the late 1940s periodic inquiries into the financing and delivery of health care services in New York City.

Our first in-depth inquiry, *A Pattern for Health Care* (1949), was performed at the request of Governor Thomas E. Dewey, and developed recommendations as to the preferred policies that the State of New York should follow in the planning and financing of hospital care in the post-World War II environment which was marked by the rapid expansion of private health insurance.

In the early 1960s the staff completed its next study, *Planning for Better Hospital Care: Report on the Hospitals and Health Agencies of the Federation of Jewish Philanthropies in New York*. The primary charge to the staff had been to assess the changed financing, demographic, and professional trends that were impacting the eleven Federation hospitals that together accounted for almost one-quarter of all inpatient care provided under voluntary auspices in New York City in an environment in which philanthropic contributions had declined from about 30 percent of total hospital revenues at the start of World War II to just 9 percent by the end of the 1950s.

A decade later saw the publication of *Urban Health Services: The Case of New York* (1971), a study that had been sponsored by the Planning Commission of the City of New York to assist it in refining its planning and policy guidelines for the future of the City's health sector. The final chapter contained fifteen specific recommendations to help the Planning Commission discharge its future responsibilities more effectively.

Shortly thereafter in cooperation with the Josiah Macy, Jr. Foundation the Eisenhower Center organized a conference on the University Medical Center and the Metropolis and subsequently (1974) published the proceedings under the same title. This was followed by a special study for Empire Blue Cross of New York, *Home Health Care: Its Role in the Changing Health Services Market* (1984).

Two years later (1986) the staff published *From Health Dollars to Health Services: New York City, 1965–1985*, which explored the sizable increases in the financing of health care over the two decades after the introduction of Medicare and Medicaid at a time when the city's population declined by about 1 million. In many respects this effort was the direct ancestor of the present volume.

The final effort that needs to be noted is *Changing U.S. Health Care: A Study of Four Metropolitan Areas*, published in 1993. This in-depth case study of the nation's four largest metropolitan centers—New York, Chicago, Houston and Los Angeles—sought to explore and assess the effects of the continuing rapid increases in health care expenditures on the quantity and quality of the medical care available to the substantial numbers of individuals who lacked adequate health insurance coverage.

If it be true, as many of us have long believed, that most health care is local, that was ample justification for focusing attention on New York City, specifically on *Improving the Health Care of the Poor: The New York City Experience*. We were pleased that the president and staff of the Robert Wood Johnson Foundation saw merit in our proposal and we wish to thank them for their support of this as well as several of our earlier research investigations into the evolving health care system of New York City.

In the course of the research the three senior authors were assisted by two former members of the Eisenhower Center staff who played key roles in the identification, collection, and analysis of critical bodies of data for which we are most grateful. They are Reshmi Siddique and Christopher Zurawsky.

The final manuscript owes its veracity to our long-time senior associate, Anna Dutka, who assumed primary responsibility for verifying the multitudinous facts and figures that gave structure and support to our argument and conclusions. Only those who have had direct experience in ferreting out the sources and assessing the validity of state and local health care data can appreciate the challenges that she faced and the success that she achieved.

Gregory Grove contributed his formidable technical skills to the treatment of quantitative data. Charles Frederick, financial and personnel officer of the Center, managed the various administrative aspects of the project with efficiency and good humor.

As has been true for many years, the skill with which Shoshana Vasheetz oversaw the preparation of successive versions of the manuscript and the production of the final draft calls for special acknowledgment and thanks.

Finally, we are indebted to Laurence Mintz of Transaction Publishers for his deft editing, patience with our compulsive reworking of the manuscript, and guidance through the toils of the production process. His participation greatly enhanced the final product; however, we alone are responsible for any errors and shortcomings that remain.

Eli Ginzberg, director
The Eisenhower Center for the
Conservation of Human Resources
Columbia University
March 1996

1

Why New York City?

Since New York City, like all American cities except for Washington D.C., is a subsidiary jurisdiction of its parent state, it is important to note at the beginning of this inquiry into the health care of the poor, several distinctive characteristics of New York State that have significantly influenced the evolution of the city's health care system. The hallmark of health policy in New York State since the early to mid-1960s has been a strong regulatory approach with stringent rules and regulations limiting the ability of public, nonprofit, or for-profit enterprises to enter and operate freely in the health care sector and/or to undertake major new capital investments. Since the early 1980s the state of New York has also determined the policies and rules governing payments for hospital care as well as authorized the imposition of surcharges on the various payers for distribution among hospitals that treat disproportionate numbers of poor people.

Three other facets of state policy are also worth noting. First, the state of New York has implemented and maintained one of the most liberal Medicaid programs of any state in the union; its expenditures per capita are about double those of California. Second, nothwithstanding this differentially high level of spending for Medicaid, the state's reimbursement rate to physicians for office visits has been kept to a minimum, currently $13. As a consequence, most physicians in private practice in New York City do not accept Medicaid patients.

Third, New York, alone among all the states that contain large cities, requires localities to pay half of the state's mandatory share of total Medicaid expenditures. Successive mayors of New York City have sought to persuade the state legislature to follow common practice and cover the nonfederal share in its entirety but so far they have had only marginal

1

success and given current and potential state budgetary deficits early relief is unlikely.

If we include New York Medical College which is located in Valhalla, Westchester County, but conducts much of its clinical training in the city, there are seven academic health centers (AHCs) that sponsor residency training programs in New York City. For more than a decade the state commissioner of health and other state officials have sought to persuade the New York City AHCs to shift their residency training emphasis from subspecialist to generalist programs (family practice, internal medicine, and pediatrics) but until a short time ago, there was relatively little response. Recently the state put another item onto its policy agenda: a significant reduction by the AHCs of the total numbers in graduate medical education (GME) programs because the cost of training comes high, about $200,000 per resident per year, and a large proportion, about half of all those who complete their training, relocate out of state.

A closely related factor: about one-third of all residents in the state whose training is paid for by Medicare are international medical graduates (IMGs), that is, graduates of foreign medical schools; in New York City the figure is close to 50 percent. Two major national leadership groups—the Council on Graduate Medical Education (COGME), an advisory body to the Congress on physician personnel, and the Association of American Medical Colleges (AAMC), the major organizational umbrella for the nation's medical colleges—have advocated limiting the number of IMGs in residency training supported by Medicare to no more than 10 percent of the annual number of graduates, approximately 16,000, from U.S. medical schools. It is uncertain what if any action the Congress will take but the odds point to a reduction in funding for IMGs in the near-middle term. If Congress should act this year (1996), the New York Health and Hospitals Corporation (HHC), which provides a high proportion of the ambulatory and inpatient care for the New York City poor, will confront a serious challenge because of its heavy dependence on IMGs for its physician staffing.

An integral factor in the financing and delivery of health care services to the city's poor is the system of "affiliation contracts" that was first developed in the early 1960s. Faced with the threatened loss of accreditation by several public hospitals, the Hospital Department contracted with local medical schools and academic health centers to assume responsibility for staffing its facilities with residents and supervisory faculty. The affiliation contracts were devised to permit the continued operation of the public hospitals that were unable to attract the requisite number of qualified housestaff and competent attending physicians from among the remaining practitioners in the low-income areas of the city where most of the municipal hospitals were located. The city has appropriated ever larger sums (about half a billion dollars in 1995) to cover the expenses incurred by these affiliation agreements.

Since the affiliation agreements with selected AHCs date back to the early 1960s, one might expect close ties to have developed between the municipal and voluntary hospital sectors. But this has not been the case. The voluntary hospitals have maintained an arm's length relationship with the city for many decades, in fact ever since the last century. This "distancing" is not difficult to explain. The voluntary sector has always had to seek philanthropic contributions to help it cover the charitable services that it provides as well as to secure needed funding for innovations and capital improvements. Closer relationships with the city would expose the voluntary hospitals to vastly increased pressures to provide more extensively for the poor than their ordinary fund-raising potential would support. Better to keep their distance. At present, however, the question must be raised whether such arm's length relations between the two hospital sectors—now complicated by the recent rapid growth of managed care and particularly Medicaid managed care—can continue much longer given the accumulating evidence of an excessive number of hospital beds; the intention of the mayor to shrink the HHC system and, if possible, to extricate the city from the direct delivery of health care services; and the explorations by leading teaching hospitals and AHCs of new alignments, consolidations, and mergers.

By all odds, the single most important development in U.S. health care policy during the last third of this century was the passage and implementation in 1965–1966 of Medicare and Medicaid. These overarching interventions in the nation's health care system form the point of departure for this study and set the framework for the analyses that follow and the "lessons for policy" that are extracted.

The first point to emphasize is that each of these programs was directed to a defined subgroup of the population. Medicare was designed to respond to the unmet needs of the elderly who faced serious difficulties in gaining broad access to the acute care system; Medicaid was passed to expand the opportunities for selected groups of the poor, in particular single mothers and their children, to obtain comprehensive services. At various intervals in the succeeding years, each program was amended for the purpose of expanding coverage, easing beneficiary contributions, or improving benefits; 1972 and 1988–89 were two periods of significant enhancement.

The objective of the Eisenhower Center staff in undertaking this inquiry into improving the health care of the New York City poor was to assess the extent to which these two new programs proved responsive to the expectations of the citizenry and presented realistic challenges to the bureaucracy charged with making them work.

The decision to examine a broad national program such as Medicare and a federal-state program such as Medicaid through the prism of their impacts on the residents of a single city—the nation's largest—requires some explanation. We started with the important premise that health care delivery is predominantly local. There were also a number of other significant factors, specific to New York City: its longstanding commitment (since the late 1920s) to provide essential health care to all citizens irrespective of their ability to pay; its bifurcated hospital system consisting of two largely independent sectors, voluntary and public, with, however, considerable overlap since the voluntary sector provides most of the physician personnel required to operate the public system. And finally there was the infusion of substantial new funding, governmental and private. Both programs were associated with new streams of funding primarily from the federal government but also from the state.

At a meeting at the New York Academy of Medicine shortly after Medicare and Medicaid were launched, the then mayor of New York, John V. Lindsay, ventured the opinion that these new sources of health care funding would assure the city a much improved budgetary outlook, since the federal and state governments would henceforth cover the steadily increasing municipal health care outlays. What this optimistic projection failed to take into account was the fact that while new sources of funding would surely become available, the demand for new services might well outpace the supply of new health care dollars, in which case the City might paradoxically find itself in a worsening budgetary position in the years ahead.

Several other factors contributed to the desirability of undertaking a detailed case study of the changes in medical care that the city's poor obtained. Scale was one. Although New York City was known to be home to large numbers of the poor, the actual size of this population was not known. Preliminary calculations indicated that the sum of Medicaid eligibles, the uninsured, and the underinsured (those whose policies would not cover a catastrophic illness) came to a grand total of 3.7 million, half of a total population of 7.4 million. Not included were most of the elderly covered by Medicare who received no Medicaid supplementation although a high proportion had incomes that fell within a range of 200 percent of the poverty level.

There was yet another reason for focusing attention on New York City. Recent government reports indicated that during the past decade the U.S. had attracted about 1 million immigrants a year, approximately 100,000 of whom established, at least temporarily, a residence in New York City. Many of these new arrivals not only lacked medical insurance, they also presented further challenges to the health care sector by virtue of their inability to speak English—at least initially.

The tendency of immigrants, many of them poor, to concentrate in selected neighborhoods close to their compatriots and others of shared race or ethnicity, themselves generally poor too, imposed further strain on the provision of effective medical services to those in need of care. Graduates of U.S. medical schools who were planning to practice in New York City—as well as those with established practices—avoided (re)locating in poorer areas of the city where the ratio of private practitioners to the population was of the order of 1 to 5,000 or even 1 to 10,000 as opposed to 1 to 500 prevailing in the more affluent areas of the city. One of the most unyielding problems in the delivery of improved health care to large concentrations of low-income populations in the city is the avoidance of these neighborhoods by U.S.-trained physicians.

Throughout the 1980s, Dr. David Axelrod, then state commissioner of health, sought to persuade both the voluntary and the municipal sectors to expand by an order of magnitude community health care centers so as to improve the access of the local poor to improved generalist care. He had relatively little success. The AHCs for the most part had other priorities such as the expansion and intensification of their efforts in biomedical research and subspecialty training; and the city of New York was operating under such constrained budgets that there was little money available to convert older facilities or build new ones to strengthen ambulatory care in low-income neighborhoods. Although New York City currently contains a number of strong community health care clinics, the scale and scope of these facilities is far more limited than those in Boston and some other metropolitan centers.

During the first two decades after World War II the city underwent a vast demographic change: 2 million of its population relocated to the suburbs and were replaced by 2 million newcomers, mostly minorities. The subsequent addition during the past decade of about 1 million immigrants helps to explain why the infrastructure for a vigorous community health care center has failed to keep pace with the need in most parts of the city.

If we turn to the question of whether and to what extent the health care services available to the New York City poor improved as the result of the new legislative interventions of Medicare and Medicaid, the answer is not simple or clear-cut, except in the case of the elderly. The rates established by the federal government to reimburse acute care hospitals and physicians for services to Medicare patients were sufficiently close to norms in private practice that the overwhelming majority of the elderly were readily accepted by virtually all hospitals and most physicians and thus were enabled to enter mainstream U.S. medical care.

After the amendments to Medicaid in 1972 that made routine nursing home care available to Medicaid-eligible patients—and many became so by the simple device of transferring assets to their relatives—the liberal reimbursement rates authorized by New York State stimulated an expansion of bed capacity. The enlarged supply facilitated admission and retention of the elderly who needed nursing home care. Still later, in 1977, the state legislature passed the Long Term Home Health Care Act (Lombardi Act), which offered many of the poor elderly an attractive alternative—the option to be cared for at home if the costs of such treatment did not exceed 75 percent of the costs of nursing home care.

A comprehensive answer to the question of how the expanded financing system contributed to improving the care available to the New York City poor over the last three decades must not fail to recognize that Medicare and Medicaid outlays were of substantial assistance to both the voluntary and the municipal hospitals in keeping abreast with the increasingly sophisticated medical technology associated with advances in biomedical R&D. Although the municipal hospitals lagged behind the voluntary sector in benefitting from the new, they would have fallen hopelessly behind had it not been for these new sources of funding.

Nevertheless, the last three decades were by no means a period in which the hospitals were totally relieved of financial concerns, particularly the HHC facilities. In 1975 the city government came within hours or days of declaring itself bankrupt and only the combined efforts of the municipal government and the trade unions with a large constituency of municipal employees together with major assists from the State of New York and (somewhat belatedly) from the federal government enabled the city to avoid default. Control and oversight of the financial affairs of the city were vested in the Municipal Assistance Corporation (MAC), a specially appointed body, until the early 1980s when the national and the local economy entered on a long cycle of expansion. The subsequent stock market crash in 1987 and its aftermath left the city's finances once again in a weakened position, forcing Mayors Dinkins and Giuliani to confront serious structural imbalances in the city's budget that were worsened by the deteriorating financial position of both the state and the federal governments.

These recurrent fiscal crises were not the only vicissitudes that the city faced in meeting the needs of the poor for more and better health care services. The 1980s saw the emergence of new, unanticipated threats that could not be ignored. First and most devastating was the invasion of the AIDS pandemic. New York City rapidly established itself as the AIDS capital of the U.S. The state commissioner of health exercised his considerable powers and influence to persuade the voluntary hospitals to assume a significant share of the responsibility for the care of AIDS patients. The HHC hospitals could not be the sole source of care.

Responding to the urgent needs of the rapidly increasing number of AIDS patients was by no means the only new challenge. There was the simultaneous emergence of various resistant strains of the tubercle bacillus with rising need for both inpatient and outpatient care in a system that since the advent of pharmaceutical treatment had all but eliminated tuberculosis beds. In addition, the radical reduction of inpatient psychiatric services generated a critical need of medical care and housing for substantial numbers of deinstitutionalized patients. The city's chronic housing dearth was exacerbated by the closure of many single-room occupancy (SRO) buildings. To complicate matters further, in the late 1980s the municipal and voluntary hospitals faced a shortage of both beds and nursing personnel. Occupancy rates soared and many hospitals, particularly those of the HHC, lacked nurses. Fortunately, both of these emergencies were resolved in the early 1990s.

There were still other political, structural, and managerial issues that affected the financing and delivery of health care services to the city's poor. Some of their more important dimensions follow:

- The bifurcated trade union structure of the voluntary and municipal hospital workforces—Local 1199 for the voluntary hospitals, District Council 37 for the municipal hospitals. Aside from these major bargaining agents, small numbers of workers are represented by other unions. As has been noted, District Council 37, under the longtime leadership of Victor Gottbaum, played a key role in helping to avert the imminent bankruptcy of the city in 1975 and subsequently assisted it to regain fiscal independence under the terms of a new labor agreement in the early 1980s.
- Periodic soundings by the political leadership in New York City and New York State of the goals, organizing principles, and collective actions (threatened or actual) of the union leadership in their drive for new members and improved wages and benefits. The vast regulatory power of the state of New York over hospital reimbursements has enabled the governor and his staff on occasion to intervene in threatened or actual strikes to wring an agreement from the parties with the promise that the costs of the settlement would be taken into consideration in the next round of rate-setting.
- Other interconnections, especially between the HHC and local politicians, that influence the operations of the public system. The HHC was established by state statute in the late 1970s to liberate the administrators of the city's health and hospital departments from the excessive control and interference of mainline city agencies. However, the loosening, much less the separation, of the two was never realized. Operating most years in a constrained budgetary environment, the mayor and his senior staff did not consider it prudent or feasible to yield much independence to the HHC. A constant source of ineffectiveness in the HHC system has been the limited authority that the HHC central administration has been willing to delegate to the directors of its member hospitals.

The interacting political, managerial, and workforce issues confronting the eleven acute care hospitals of the HHC have been further complicated by the power of local political leaders to determine appointments and promotions when openings occur in their respective neighborhood institutions. Inasmuch as a large HHC hospital is the principal employer in a neighborhood that is short of jobs, especially decent jobs with reasonable pay and benefits, the powerful role of local political chiefs in the selection and advancement of hospital personnel is a fact of life that goes far to explain many of the frustrations experienced even by capable hospital directors in their attempts to provide quality care within the limits of the resources available to them.

The chapters that follow have sought to identify, analyze, and evaluate these interactions over the last three decades as they affected the results of the much expanded annual outlays for health care services in New York City, which rose from approximately $20 to $44 billion in constant dollars in a period when the city's population declined by about a half million, or some 6 percent. Another notable observation: in per capita expenditures for health care (around $6,000) New York City leads the nation by approximately 50 percent. This differential has remained more or less constant throughout the thirty-year period we have covered in our evaluation.

Given the soaring rate of health care spending, it is striking that there exists no instrumentality in the voluntary or public sector, at the city or state level, that has the charge, resources, and public trust to monitor developments in the financing and delivery of health care services to the people of New York City, poor and nonpoor alike. The arm's length posture of the voluntary sector with respect to conjoint action on health issues with the municipal government doubtless has contributed to the absence of any broad public oversight of these vast annual health care outlays. The press is aroused periodically by the occurrence of an unnecessary death referable to some error of omission or commission. The voluntary sector sponsors various organizations that raise funds for the purpose of influencing the direction of public policies that may affect their mission and goals. And the universities conduct restricted or broader programs of research and evaluation. No institution, however, even pretends to maintain oversight of changes in the total system, much less assess future changes that might lead to improved outcomes.

Nevertheless there is reason to believe that the decade ahead will differ in many respects from the three decades that preceded it. Each of the public payers for health care services in New York City—the federal, state, and municipal governments—is in the clutches of a budgetary crisis that has little likelihood of early resolution. Since these three payers account for more than half of the total outlays for health care in New York City, the future cannot be simply a projection of the past.

There is additional support for the likelihood of significant changes in the decade ahead. In 1991, the New York State legislature mandated the enrollment of increasing numbers of Medicaid beneficiaries in managed care plans and the intervening years have seen considerable action to speed this goal. Although the effort has been interrupted because of improprieties and irregularities in enrollment practices, once these difficulties have been resolved the growth of managed care plans will resume and probably accelerate.

Governor Pataki has received the report of a panel headed by the state commissioner of health recommending termination of the New York Prospective Hospital Reimbursement Methodology (NYPHRM), the long ensconced hospital reimbursement regulatory apparatus, when the current enabling legislation expires on June 30, 1996. The system is likely to be replaced by direct price negotiations between payers and the providers of care. This revision, which is likely to be approved by the state legislature, although not without adjustments and refinements, will radically alter the principles that have shaped hospital reimbursements since the early 1980s.

Finally, there is mounting evidence of profound changes in the environment and operations of the voluntary sector equal to or greater than those identified above. A recently published volume, *Tomorrow's Hospital: A Look to the 21st Century* (Ginzberg, Yale University Press, 1996), sets out some of the radical changes that are likely to alter and circumscribe the central role that the acute care hospital has played in the provision of health care to the American people since the end of World War II. Among the issues that will be addressed in the years immediately ahead are the potential and limitations of managed care plans to moderate health expenditures and at the same time satisfy the majority of Americans with the quantity and quality of care that they deliver. The future trend in the number of uninsured Americans is uncertain, and it is not clear how the public will respond should that figure rise to an intolerable level.

The experience of New York City as it sought to broaden and improve the health care services to the poor during the past three decades should prove instructive for the city and the nation as they face the even more dynamic period ahead.

2

The Changing Health Care Delivery System

Since the subject of our study is the poor of New York City, we need to clarify at the outset precisely whom the term "the poor" encompasses. Our principal interest is how people with constrained access to health care receive services and while this is primarily a low-income population, it may include individuals who do not fall below the federal poverty standard. Within this definition, we include persons on Medicaid, persons without health insurance, and persons who are underinsured, that is, whose benefits fall short of their needs in range and/or volume. We also include people who may have monetary assets or insurance coverage but who are disadvantaged racially, ethnically, or linguistically. In New York City this is not a negligible group. There are 2 million Medicaid-eligible individuals and an estimated 1.5 million uninsured living within the city limits. Assuming an additional 500,000 people who are underinsured or otherwise disadvantaged, the group we are looking at amounts to almost 50 percent of the total city population.

Much has been made of the concept that the "market" is now reforming the health care system in New York City (and across the nation), but this is neither correct in the economic sense nor valid in terms of the poor. With over 50 percent of health care costs funded directly by federal, state, and local government, and with additional costs mediated through tax policy, it is simply wrong to talk about the dominating role of the market. The United States has long had a pluralistic health care system in which government and the private sector have both been involved in the financing and operation of health care delivery. If anything, the amount of public funding for health care has been increasing at the expense of private spending. Moreover, for those classified as poor, access to care is almost completely mediated through public finance. This is especially true in New York City where there is not only substantial

Medicaid and Medicare spending, but also a large public hospital system, tax-exempt financing of private hospitals and clinics, and a state-run hospital reimbursement system with revenue redistribution for uncompensated care. Almost all commercial managed care plans have until recently avoided enrolling the poor, and those that now service the Medicaid managed care population are dependent on public dollars. In the context of the present study, which is focused on New York City and more particularly on policy directions for improving the health care of the urban poor, reliance on market-based reforms raises a large number of questions, specifically, the future rate of growth of the managed care plans; the ability of the plans to attract and retain a significant proportion of the specialists practicing in New York City and to satisfy the city's sophisticated consumers; and whether the managed care plans will develop the requisite capabilities to respond to the large numbers of poor patients, many of whom are chronically ill or disabled.

Consider the following challenges to the oversimplified view that "the market" will sooner or later set everything right within our health care system. Basic to the workings of a market economy are a continuing flow of upstream investments that are required to maintain the effectiveness of the health delivery system, investments involving the education and training of physicians and other health professionals; the funding and performance of biomedical research, the foundation for the significant advances in knowledge and technique related to medical diagnosis and treatment; and the construction, maintenance, and continued upgrading of hospitals and other critical facilities where physicians, other health professionals, technicians, and support staff can effectively treat the most seriously injured and ill patients.

Since most of the funding required for medical education, biomedical research, and major treatment centers has been provided by government with a substantial assist from philanthropy, profit-seeking dollars play relatively minor roles, principally in the financing of for-profit hospital chains and managed care plans, and the development and marketing of sophisticated medical equipment and pharmaceuticals. All of the latter, it must be recalled, are greatly dependent on basic biomedical research which up to the present has been financed overwhelmingly by the federal government.

It was not preordained that government should assume the leadership in upstream biomedical investments nor is there reason to assume that it must maintain this role in perpetuity. The burden of proof, however, is on the advocates of the market to provide the scenario indicating how and why the market-oriented, profit-seeking sector will be motivated/impelled to replace government as the principal investor in the capital infrastructure. Absent such a persuasive scenario backed by implementing actions, it makes more sense to assume that government's role will change slowly, if at all. This is further reason to continue to use the pluralistic model rather than the market model in assessing the U.S. health care system and exploring ways in which it can be made more efficient and responsive to the needs of all Americans.

Although the point is often made by critics of our health care system that the United States is the only large, advanced nation that does not provide universal health care coverage for its citizens, this does not imply that the sizable number of the poor do not have access to essential care. The public and private providers of health care have long made services available to patients who are unable to pay in part or in full for their care. By custom and increasingly by law, the poor who turn to hospitals that have emergency rooms (which means virtually all hospitals in urban areas) and clinics are able to obtain essential care, though their care—ambulatory or inpatient—is seldom the equivalent of that available to persons with good insurance coverage. With no regular source of care, they frequently seek treatment too late and the care they receive is not of the quality obtained by those who have an ongoing relationship with their physician.

Although four out of every five Americans live in a metropolitan area, the location of hospitals, clinics, and physician offices are significant determinants of the quantity and quality of the services that individuals seek and obtain. This helps to explain the concern of all levels of government with the "locational" aspects of health care, particularly the ability of low-income urban neighborhoods (as well as outlying rural areas) to attract and retain adequate numbers of physicians and other essential health personnel. Although all levels of government have addressed the locational aspects of health care delivery repeatedly since the passage of the Hill-Burton Act in 1946 (and even before at state and local levels), given a society predicated on freedom of work and residence, the U.S. has experienced only limited success in persuading physicians to practice, even for a specified number of years, among underserved populations. The simplistic explanation is that government has not been willing to offer sufficiently attractive incentives in the form of educational debt forgiveness, salaries, and bonuses. But there is more to the story. Well-trained physicians will not willingly agree to practice in neighborhoods where the medical infrastructure does not permit them to utilize the skills that they have laboriously acquired during a lengthy period (seven to ten years or more) of professional education and training. Moreover, race— the fact that most physicians are white while most of the urban poor are not—is a major factor in the shortfall of private medical care in inner-city areas that will not change quickly, if at all, even if universal health insurance coverage is enacted.

There is another aspect to the issue of location in relation to the market model of health care. Little attention has been paid to the fact that most medical care is a local service, an important consideration in terms of the future structure of health care delivery to the American people. Some years ago, a sophisticated student of the American health care system, Dr. Paul Ellwood, looked forward to the time that a dozen or so mega-corporations would deliver most, if not all, of the nation's health care. This hypothesis has been revived in the wake of recent developments: many experts predict that the rapidly proliferating managed care plans will eventually be reduced in number to no more than three or so for each of the larger metropolitan areas.

While this forecast may turn out to be correct, it is surely premature because, as suggested earlier, the anticipated growth and long-term survival of the managed care plans have yet to be demonstrated; the dominance of the locational factor in all health delivery systems is a major consideration; and there is little or no evidence that managed care plans will be able to deal effectively with "the poor" who account for about one in three Americans.

The foregoing analysis of the contemporary U.S. health care system can be summarized along the following axes:

- The outstanding characteristic of the U.S. health care system, surely in the mid-1990s, is its pluralism. Unlike most other advanced countries where government accounts on average for between 75 and 85 percent of total health care outlays, the ratio of governmental to nongovernmental spending in the United States is more nearly 50–50. With government currently the immediate source for half of all outlays, it is clearly inappropriate, in fact simply wrong, to place the current health care system in the framework of "the market." This is not to say that a more dominant market role

might not develop in the years and decades ahead, but the odds—despite
the growth of managed care plans—are that government will play an even
larger role as the payer of health care dollars.

- Although universal health care has not been adopted in the United States,
  all Americans have access to essential care through the emergency rooms
  and clinics of the nation's public and voluntary hospitals. This statement
  does not mean—or even imply—that the poor who turn to the hospital for
  ambulatory or inpatient care receive the same amount and quality of care
  as would be available to a well-insured person from his personal physician
  and from the voluntary hospital(s) to which he or she was admitted.

- With one out of every seven dollars of gross domestic product (GDP) being
  spent in the health care sector and with the sector accounting for about 10
  million workers (or over 8 percent of the nation's employed labor force),
  the stakes are high for the average American who sees his or her physician
  four or five times a year; and even higher for the one in eight who are
  hospitalized. The stakes are also high for the members of the principal
  provider groups—in particular, hospitals, physicians, other health care and
  support personnel, health insurance companies, medical schools and academic health centers (AHCs), pharmaceutical and medical supply companies, and others.

- Improving the health care of New York City's poor requires us to examine
  carefully the expansionary forces that affected New York City's pluralistic
  health care system since 1960, the period immediately preceding the passage of Medicare and Medicaid; assess the aims and intent of the major
  policies that were adopted and the extent to which each was realized, with
  particular reference to the health care of the city's poor. The conclusions,
  however tentative, drawn from this analysis, can help to inform the challenge that confronts all of the nation's cities.

The best way to delineate the pluralism of New York City's health
care delivery system is to consider briefly how the poor obtain access to
care, focusing primarily on the provider institutions, from private practitioners to the public and voluntary hospital systems.

Sources of Medical Care for the Poor in New York City

Having defined the poor as those with restricted access to medical
care facilities and services, we will examine the sources of care that they
use. In some ways, the most remarkable feature of this list is how similar
the services are to those the nonpoor tend to use. The essential difference
between the two is in the availability of services and the amenities to
which the nonpoor have access and the poor do not.

TABLE 2.1
Sources of Medical Care in New York City

Site	Use by the Nonpoor	Use by the Poor
Private MD office	X	
Public medical clinic		X
Medicaid Mill		X
Hospital-operated clinic		X
OPD		X
ER	X	X
Private hospital	X	X
Public hospital		X
School health program		X
Union health clinic	X	

There are other differences in access to care between the poor and the nonpoor. For one thing, the poor enrolled in Medicaid may receive their nonhospital based ambulatory care from physicians who are predominantly international medical graduates (IMGs). Almost 40 percent of the physicians in New York City are IMGs who are far more likely to accept Medicaid as a form of payment than USMGs. The larger proportion of Medicaid enrollees receive their ambulatory care at the emergency rooms and clinics of the HHC or voluntary hospitals. It is important to note that the high utilization of institutionally based ambulatory services in New York City is a function of the small number of private physicians who participate in the Medicaid program and of the higher reimbursement rates offered by Medicaid to hospitals and clinics. This revenue makes Medicaid-eligibles desirable patients. Under the New York Prospective Hospital Reimbursement Methodology (NYPHRM) hospital payment system, inpatient Medicaid rates are set at the same level as Blue Cross rates, while hospitals receive an all-inclusive fee for outpatient and ER visits. This fee is capped at $67.50 for OPD services and $92.50 for ER services. However, the inclusion of payments for capital costs and GME can greatly increase hospital revenues.

One result of this push-pull cost inflation has been recent attempts by the state to reduce Medicaid costs by eliminating institutionally provided ambulatory care through the greater use of managed primary care services. Until recently, only small numbers of Medicaid patients were enrolled in the Health Insurance Plan, the largest and oldest HMO in the city or in the Bronx Health Plan that was established in the mid-1980s to cater specifically to Medicaid enrollees in several locations in the Bronx.

Following the passage of the Medicaid Managed Care Act by the state legislature in 1991, a major new modality was introduced specifically aimed at the Medicaid population. The legislature decided that selected counties in New York State, including the 5 counties comprising New York City, had to enroll in managed care plans at least 50 percent of all Medicaid beneficiaries by the end of 1997 in the belief that this would result in cost savings for the state (and city) and would expand and improve the health care services available to the poor by increasing their access to preventive services. Faced with a severe budgetary deficit, the newly elected Governor Pataki shortly after assuming office in January 1995 committed the state of New York to a much accelerated schedule of enrollments and submitted to the Health Care Financing Administration (HCFA) a proposal for a federal waiver that would permit compulsory enrollment of the Medicaid population in managed care plans. As of July 1996, HCFA has not yet acted on New York State's waiver request.

Another source of ambulatory care for the city's Medicaid population are the freestanding D and T (diagnostic and treatment) centers that provide a considerable volume of services to the residents of low-income neighborhoods. Most of these are community health centers funded by the federal government, either original OEO clinics or Urban Health Initiative (Section 330) clinics. A small number are union- or company-sponsored health clinics with a restricted clientele. Ten percent of the ambulatory care visits made by Medicaid patients are to a community health clinic.

While hospitals have enjoyed the revenues produced by ambulatory visits from the Medicaid population, this income stream is offset by increasing costs of providing care and by the large number of noninsured patients for whom the hospitals are not reimbursed. Most hospitals have attempted to establish off-site (and hence lower cost) clinics in which to handle nonemergency, that is, primary care services.

Several of the city's leading AHCs—in particular Einstein-Montefiore and Columbia-Presbyterian—have been involved for longer or shorter periods of time in operating neighborhood health care delivery systems that are predicated on cooperative arrangements with selected physicians who practice in the neighborhood and who receive back-up support from the cooperating AHC. The Presbyterian Hospital, for example, created the Ambulatory Care Network Corporation (ACNC) an independent corporation consisting of the Vanderbilt Clinic (the outpatient department of Presbyterian) and a number of off-site clinics as a mechanism to reduce the cost of outpatient care at Vanderbilt Clinic by eliminating hospital-based overhead, and to capture higher revenues than a hospital-based ambulatory care center could get directly through Medicaid. Since its inception in the early 1980s, the ACNC has received an experimental Medicaid reimbursement rate that exceeds the hospital-based rate for caring for similar types of patients.

Lutheran Hospital, in southwest Brooklyn, has pioneered over many years in developing a growing network of ambulatory care clinics to meet the needs of the large number of previous and newly settled low-income groups in the area, a high proportion of whom are on Medicaid.

Still another illustration of the outreach activities undertaken by selected voluntary hospitals in response to the unmet health care needs of the poor is the widely recognized Methadone Maintenance Treatment Program (MMTP) for heroin addicts that Beth Israel Medical Center launched in 1965. It has expanded continuously, serving about 8,000 enrollees per year in 1995.

Without pretending to be an inclusive inventory of the diverse opportunities for the city's poor to obtain access to ambulatory care services, note must also be taken of the following: the well-baby clinics operated by the city's Department of Health which are currently being transferred to the HHC; school health programs which were included in the service infrastructure of most of the city's public schools up to the city's fiscal crisis of 1975 (the program was radically reduced as the Department of Health suffered severe reductions in its subsequent budgets, with the result that no more than one in five schools had a program in operation at the end of 1994).

To continue: both the city and the voluntary sector provide limited amounts of health care services to adults and children who make use of the shelters for the homeless. Most of the Headstart programs provide a limited volume of health services for their enrollees and some health care education for parents. There are also a considerable number of specialized health care clinics located throughout the city that provide a range of specialized services (evaluation and treatment) to the poor: family planning, mental health, alcohol and drug abuse, rehabilitation, the blind, and many others.

The large numbers of the poor who are not eligible for Medicaid or who, if eligible, have not enrolled must rely in the first instance on the emergency rooms and clinics of the HHC hospitals, and, depending on location or the urgency of their condition, on the ambulatory care facilities of nearby voluntary hospitals. Many of the poor who lack Medicaid coverage quickly learn that the HHC hospitals recognize their responsibility to treat them and that most voluntary hospitals, some subtly and others less subtly, induce them to seek their care in the nearby public institutions. This practice of "patient-dumping" (as it is known in other parts of the country) has gone on for so long in New York City that it has become an institutionalized and recognized pattern of patient transfer. This interplay is particularly pervasive in the case of private hospitals that are located adjacent or proximate to public hospitals; it is somewhat more difficult when the hospitals are not contiguous. Currently Medicaid accounts for 45 percent of all outpatient visits to voluntary and HHC facilities and for 40 percent of emergency room visits in HHC facilities and 34 percent in voluntary hospitals.

When it comes to inpatient acute care, the utilization patterns are different. As noted earlier, most of the non-Medicaid poor seek and receive care in HHC hospitals. While the HHC hospitals also admit large numbers of Medicaid patients for inpatient treatment, the majority are cared for in voluntary hospitals.

We will consider briefly the infrastructure for long-term care consisting of chronic care hospitals, nursing homes, and home care. The city operates two hospitals on Roosevelt Island in the East River for patients requiring long-term care. There are a total of 166 licensed nursing homes throughout the five boroughs under voluntary or for-profit auspices. A high proportion of all nursing home patients are enrolled in Medicaid, the majority at the time of admission, others after they have "spent down" to meet the asset criteria of the program.

The Long Term Home Health Care Act (Lombardi Act), passed by the state legislature in 1977, permitted Medicaid to offer nursing home-eligible patients the option to be treated at home if the cost would not exceed 75 percent of the average cost of care in a nursing home. Given the shortage of nursing home beds, New York City took the lead in responding to this opportunity to care for large numbers of the disabled and the elderly in their homes. At the end of 1994 enrollment in the Medicaid home care program in New York City totaled around 62,000.

An overview of the pluralistic nature of the health care system in New York City cannot overlook the presence of hospitals and both on- and off-site clinics run by the federal government and the state of New York, which cater to specific groups of patients and/or medical conditions. There are three Veterans Administration facilities, one each in the boroughs of the Bronx, Brooklyn, and Manhattan, which provide both inpatient and ambulatory care.

The state of New York operates one acute care teaching hospital in connection with its Downstate Medical School in Brooklyn. In addition, the state provides drug rehabilitation services and other selected specialized services.

To delineate all the dimensions of the pluralism that characterizes the access of the city's poor to health care services, it is necessary also to assess the payments that are made to the provider institutions as well as the flow of other funds that determine their respective scale of operations. The increasing funding flows that continue to have such a pronounced effect on the provision of health care to the city's poor will be the subject of the next chapter.

By way of preliminary summary, the pluralism of the health services delivery system in New York City, with special reference to those agencies and institutions directly involved in providing services to the Medicaid and uninsured populations, is demonstrated by the following major groups and subgroups differentiated by type and range of services and the sectors that sponsor them—public, nonprofit or for-profit.

Public Sector

New York City

HHC hospitals and clinics
- Major providers of inpatient and ambulatory care for both Medicaid and the uninsured.
- Two hospitals for Medicaid and indigent patients requiring long-term inpatient care.

Department of Health (DOH)
- Maternal and well-baby clinics in low-income areas. These clinics are now being transferred to the HHC.

- Prior to the fiscal crisis of 1975, DOH operated an extended network of school health services. These activities were radically reduced until the late 1980s when a modest, continuing expansion began.
- The DOH also is responsible for various specialized programs such as the delivery of services to persons in public shelters, patients suffering from active tuberculosis, and a number of others.

Human Resources Administration (HRA)
- HRA has oversight of the Medicaid home care program with expenditures in 1994 of about $1.4 billion for 62,000 users.

New York State

The Department of Social Services (DOSS)
- Responsible for meeting the targets set by the state of New York for the enrollment of Medicaid enrollees in managed care plans and for ensuring that the plans meet state standards with respect to access and quality of services.
- SUNY Health Science Center at Brooklyn and University Hospital of Brooklyn
- Department of Health
- New York Substance Abuse Facilities

Federal Government

Veterans Administration Hospitals
- Manhattan
- Brooklyn
- Bronx

Non-Profit Sector

Academic Health Centers (AHCs)
- Five AHCs in Manhattan and in the Bronx and New York Medical College located in Valhalla (Westchester County) that supervise residency training programs at several affiliated hospitals, public and private, in New York City.
- The principal teaching hospital and the affiliated teaching hospitals of the six private AHCs that sponsor residency training programs and also provide extensive ambulatory and inpatient care to Medicaid and uninsured patients.
- Community partnerships of the AHCs with clinics and physicians in low-income neighborhoods aimed at providing more and better access to ambulatory care in the absence of an adequate number of competent local practitioners.

Free-standing community health clinics under neighborhood sponsorship and leadership that provide a broader or narrower range of preventive, diagnostic, and therapeutic services for the poor and near-poor, often in association with nearby community hospitals to which they refer their more seriously ill or injured patients.

HMOs
- The Health Insurance Plan of New York (HIP) established in 1944 and the Bronx Health Plan established in 1994–95 that had enrolled Medicaid beneficiaries prior to the passage in 1991 of the Medicaid Managed Care Act. Subsequent expansion of Medicaid enrollments.

Nursing homes that admit limited numbers of Medicaid enrollees and private pay patients who spend down to Medicaid eligibility.

The Visiting Nurse Association and other non-profit home care organizations that provide a range of medical services for the homebound.

For-Profit

- Local private practitioners, mostly members of group practices in low-income neighborhoods, from whom a considerable number of Medicaid enrollees and uninsured persons obtain routine medical care.
- For-profit managed care plans that have recruited since 1991 growing numbers of Medicaid enrollees on a voluntary or mandated basis.
- For-profit nursing homes that admit restricted numbers of Medicaid patients and also continue to treat private paying patients who have spent down to become Medicaid-eligible.
- For-profit home health care organizations that have proliferated in recent years. This has become the fastest growing sector of health care delivery, providing services ranging from sophisticated high-tech procedures to supportive services for the frail and elderly that enable them to remain in their own homes.

It is important to note that a similar pluralism characterizes the delivery of health care services to the non-poor, those New Yorkers with good health insurance coverage.

3

Cascade of Dollars

This chapter will review in detail the major changes in the dollar flows into the health care system of New York City between 1965, the year that Medicare and Medicaid were enacted, and 1994, with the caveat that the financial data sets for cities and states are neither as complete nor as consistent as one would wish. However, reasonable estimates can be made from the data that are available for most, if not all, categories.

A good way to begin is to set the account of the dollar flows into New York City in the broader context of the total national health care outlays or, more conventionally, total *personal* health care outlays, a figure that is 10 to 12 percent lower since it excludes research and capital funding.

On the basis of painstaking data collection and analysis, Nora Piore and her colleagues, Purlaine Lieberman and James Linnane, calculated that in 1966, the onset of Medicare and Medicaid, New York City's total expenditures for personal health care services amounted to $2.5 billion. This figure was constructed from data for the seven critical categories of personal health care expenditure: hospital care, physicians' services, dentists' services, nursing home care, drugs, other professional services and appliances, and "other health services." The report differentiated the contributions of private and public spending, the latter disaggregated by level of government—local, state, and federal.

To view the spending for New York City in perspective, we will present comparable figures for the nation's health expenditures in 1965 and subsequent sentinel years in the mid-1970s, 1980s, and 1990s.

In 1965, personal health care expenditures in the U.S. amounted to $35.6 billion, $184 per capita for a population of 194.3 million. New York City with almost 8 million residents (including some non-New Yorkers who obtained care in the city) spent a total of $2.5 billion for health care, something over $300 per person, more than half again as much as the national average.

Although there are as yet no firm figures for New York City's total health care spending in 1994, the Eisenhower Center staff has estimated that a reasonable working number would be $44 billion, an amount that informed state officials in Albany found acceptable. Of course, the figures for 1965 cannot be compared directly with those for 1994. Two adjustments must be made: one for the depreciation of the dollar, as indicated by the eightfold rise in the medical consumer price index over the intervening three decades, the other for an increase of about one-third in the total population of the U.S. at the same time that the New York City population declined by over 7 percent.

Ideally, further correction should be made for the changing numbers and proportions of persons over seventy-five in the populations of both the city and the nation since this older cohort utilizes a disproportionate volume of health care services relative to the population under sixty-five. Between 1980 and 1990, the number of individuals age seventy-five and over nationwide increased from 10 million to 13 million (about 30 percent); in New York City from 378,000 to 413,000 (over 9 percent).

Correcting for inflation and population growth, but not for age, provides the following comparative figures:

TABLE 3.1
Personal Health Care Spending in the United States and New York City:
1965, 1994
(in current and constant* dollars)

	United States		New York City	
	Current	Constant	Current	Constant
1965				
Total (billions)	$35.6	141.3	2.5	9.9
per capita	184.0	727.0	318.0	1262.0
1994				
Total (billions)	832.5	394.5	44.0	20.9
per capita	3198.0	1516.0	6027.0	2827.0

*1982 – 84 = 100

Sources: New York City, Piore
   United States, Statistical Abstract of the United States 1995; National Health Expenditure Projections, 1994–2005. Health Care Financing Review, Summer 1995.

Even after allowing for changes in both the value of the dollar and the size of the population, it is clear that the last three decades have seen a sharp rise in the funds flowing into the health care sector, both in the nation as a whole and particularly in New York City. Over the thirty-year span per capita expenditures in real health dollars doubled in the nation and more than doubled in New York City. New York City's expenditure level was more than half again as high as the national average at the end of the three decades.

Much has been made of the fact that health care expenditures over these three decades increased much more rapidly than the gross domestic product (GDP). With national health care spending in 1965 just under 6 percent of GDP, it rose to 13.9 percent in 1994 (and was estimated at 14.2 percent for 1995). The contribution of health care spending to the gross product of New York City has increased at the national rate.

By way of introduction to the analysis of the changes in spending that occurred during each of the last three decades in New York City, we will examine the national trends with respect to such critical factors as the total rate of expenditures and the principal sources of funding in both the private and public sectors.

In 1965, the breakdown of payments for personal health services revealed that most expenditures were covered out-of-pocket by consumers ($19 billion out of the total of $35.6 billion), followed by insurance ($8.7 billion) and governmental outlays (federal, state and local combined, $7.3 billion). In 1975, the following shifts were found in the national expenditure pattern: out-of-pocket payments had increased to $38.5 billion (of a total of $116.2 billion), double what they had been a decade earlier. Private insurance payments had increased more than threefold to $29.9 billion. The truly striking change, however, was in spending by the public sector which rose about sixfold, from $7.3 billion to $45.3 billion.

From a national perspective, the initial period of Medicare and Medicaid implementation (1966 to 1975) saw rapid growth in total spending, the most rapid reflecting public outlays that rose from roughly 20 percent of the total in 1965 to 39 percent of a much larger total a decade later. Another way to view the decade's changes is to emphasize the rapid decline in the proportion of out-of-pocket payments, while the share of insurance premiums remained more or less constant and governmental outlays increased dramatically.

Expenditures in New York City over the same decade can be summarized as follows: In the base year (1966) private sector payments accounted for 71 percent of the total, a few percentage points lower than the national average. Public sector expenditures came to 29 percent with the city contributing 45 percent of the total governmental share, followed by the state (37 percent) and the federal government a distant third (18 percent).

By 1976 the pattern was vastly different. While private sector expenditures had increased by 117 percent over the decade, public sector spending soared by about $4 billion over its total outlays of slightly above $700 million in 1996—a rise of more than 637 percent! Although the city and state outlays had each increased over this ten-year period from somewhat above and somewhat below $300 million respectively in 1966 to approximately $1.1 billion in 1976, the federal government outlays rocketed from $133 million to $2.28 billion. The most important change in New York City health care expenditures during the decade reflected the explosive growth in federal spending. In the base year 1966, the federal contribution amounted to under 3.5 percent of total New York City spending for health care; in the mid-1970s it rose to just under 30 percent of the total which was almost four times larger in current dollars.

The predominant shares of the approximately $6 billion of new health care expenditures during the course of the decade went to hospitals, 49 percent; physicians, 18 percent; and nursing homes, 11 percent. Seven percent of the increase went for drugs and 5 percent for dental services. The largest relative change was the increase in the proportion of health care expenditures for nursing homes that more than doubled from 4 percent to 9 percent.

Hospitals that accounted for 48 percent of total expenditures in 1976, up from 45 percent a decade earlier, were by far the principal beneficiaries of increased total and public outlays for health care services. In 1966, total hospital expenditures amounted to just under $900 million with public hospitals accounting for 42 percent, private sector hospitals for 58 percent. A decade later hospital outlays were slightly in excess of $3.3 billion. Of the $2.4 billion new dollars flowing into hospital care in New York City over the decade, $1.9 billion, or 80 percent of all of the new dollars, represented payments for Medicare and Medicaid patients, programs that had first been implemented in 1966.

Several other observations of interest can be extracted from the experience of the substantially enlarged funding that followed the introduction of Medicare and Medicaid, with a particular focus on hospitals and the impact of the new programs on the voluntary and public hospitals in New York City. For the decade as a whole, the total spending by Medicaid slightly exceeded that of Medicare; in most years the difference was within 5 percentage points with Medicaid the largest payer for hospital care. At the end of the decade, New York City's municipal hospitals received a combined total of about $600 million in revenue from the two programs which accounted for about 85 percent of the total increase in their revenues, the predominant amount coming from Medicaid.

The voluntary sector hospitals had a fourfold increase in revenues over the decade, of which Medicaid contributed $482 million and Medicare $750 million. Hidden within these totals are the following interesting details: the voluntary hospitals received slightly more in payments from Medicaid than the public hospitals; however, the real difference between the two reflected the much larger Medicare payments made to the voluntary hospitals, $750 million in 1976 compared to a mere $132 million for the municipal hospitals.

The most striking effect of the foregoing was to reduce the proportion of private funds for voluntary hospitals from 84 percent at the beginning of the decade to 41 percent at the end. The magnitude of these additional public monies flowing into the voluntary hospitals had important consequences for their long-term strategies and tactics that will be explored in subsequent chapters. At this point, one critical consequence will be mentioned: prior to the passage of Medicare and Medicaid, the trustees and staffs of voluntary hospitals were seriously constrained when it came to expansions and innovations which were limited by their available philanthropic dollars—endowment and current giving. By the mid-1970s they had entered a new era when many of their previous charity and part-pay patients had been converted into patients whose hospital costs were paid in full, with an add-on for capital depreciation by government. The hospitals were now operating in an environment in which the more they spent, the more they were reimbursed. Over 90 percent of their inpatients were covered by third party payers, in the first instance government, secondly private insurance.

To summarize the first of the dynamic three decades after the passage of Medicare and Medicaid in 1965: The new legislation made the U.S. Treasury for the first time a major source of funding for health care and also led to a sizable increase in funding by the states, and a much more modest increase by local government. Private sector funding also increased primarily as a result of additional spending by private insurance. The out-of-pocket expenditures by households doubled in dollar amount, but as a percentage of the total underwent a significant decline.

Funding for health care services in New York City during the first post-Medicare/Medicaid decade followed national trends, with, however, above-average spending for Medicaid reflecting the more liberal eligibility standards and benefit packages of the state and the city. For both the U.S. and New York City, the most striking changes were reflected in the vastly improved financial position of the hospital sector, particularly the voluntary hospitals that were paid cost-plus for treating a large number of patients who previously had paid nothing or met only part of their bills.

During the second post-Medicare/Medicaid decade, from 1975 to the mid-1980s, the flow of funding in the health care sector for the U.S. as a whole followed the trend of the preceding period. Personal health care expenditures increased in current dollars some 3.2-fold for the decade.

Expenditures in New York City during the second part of the 1970s and the first part of the 1980s (1976 to 1985) lagged behind the national trends. The principal explanation for the deceleration in the city's health care outlays was the tightening in the city's budget following the fiscal crisis of 1975 that continued until the early 1980s and a concomitant constriction in the state's Medicaid program, particularly in the number of enrollees.

The estimates of personal health care spending for 1976 reported in the Piore study and in the United Hospital Fund study for 1985 provide us with the basic data to trace what happened in New York City during the intervening ten years, both with respect to total spending and with respect to the distribution of the funds among the principal providers of health care.

The United Hospital Fund (UHF) figures for health care spending in the city for 1985 show a total of just under $17 billion as against expenditures of $8.3 billion for 1976, calculated by Piore and colleagues, or just over a doubling. However, as noted above, the increase in national expenditures for the same decade was 3.2-fold or more than half again as much in terms of current dollars.

Since the nation gained some 11 percent in population over the decade while the city population remained within 1 percent of what it had been, the per capita changes in expenditures should reflect these contrasting trends. On a per capita basis New York City still lagged the national increase but the difference was more modest. Figures for total expenditures indicate a 50 percent more rapid rate of increase for the U.S. than for New York City; per capita expenditures nationwide rose 150 percent, in the city 126 percent.

In 1976, of the $8.3 billion of total expenditures for health care in New York City, the public sector accounted for $4.6 billion (55 percent), the private sector for 3.7 billion (45 percent). A decade later the shares of the two sectors were virtually unchanged, with public outlays amounting to $9.2 billion (54 percent) and private sector funding $7.8 billion (46 percent) out of a total of $17 billion.

During this decade of relatively more constrained funding, there were some significant changes in the respective shares of the total dollar flows received by the principal providers—hospitals, physicians, and nursing homes—that together accounted for about four of every five health care dollars. In both years (1976 and 1985) the hospitals received 48 percent of all health care dollars. Somewhat unexpectedly, the share of nursing home care that had more than doubled in the first post-Medicare/Medicaid era remained constant in the second decade, about 9 percent of total spending. Physician services rose from 20 percent of total spending in 1976 to 21.5 percent in 1985. With the exception of "other personal health care," whose share dropped from 7 percent to slightly over 5 percent, all the other components ended the decade with approximately the same shares (within 1 percent) that they had had at the beginning.

Turning to the funding sources for the various health care providers during the course of the second decade, it is noteworthy that the contribution of private dollars to total hospital revenues increased from around 28 percent to 32 percent, reflecting the growth of private health insurance.

With respect to nursing home care, public dollars played an even more prominent role at the end than at the beginning of the decade, rising from around 81 percent to 86 percent of total revenues. As for physician earnings, the share of public dollars declined modestly, from 34 percent in 1976 to 30 percent ten years later.

Despite the fiscal crisis, the proportion of public dollars, just under 55 percent of all funds allocated to the health care system in 1976, remained virtually unchanged (54 percent) in the following decade. This was a function, in the first instance, of the dominant role of federal dollars and secondarily, of the volume of state dollars relative to city dollars.

This brings us to the third post-Medicare/Medicaid decade, 1986 to 1994. Although national health accounts through 1994 have been published, detailed expenditure data sets for the city comparable to those developed for the preceding two decades by the Piore-UHF studies do not exist for this most recent period. However, the following analyses of aggregate data may be useful indicators of major trends and relationships.

In the decade between 1986 and the end of 1994 national personal health care expenditures increased from $398 billion to over $832 billion. (Estimates for 1995 indicate a rise to $898 billion.) Based on a population of 260 million, this amounts to a per capita outlay in 1994 of $3450 in contrast to $1594 in 1986, for an increase of 115 percent over the nine year period, not substantially different from the per capita increase of 127 percent in the nine years from 1977 to 1985.

The similarity ends, however, once one recalls that the earlier period included years of very rapid inflation as opposed to the slower rate of inflation in the more recent decade. To be specific: in 1977 the medical care consumer price index stood at 57; by 1985 it had advanced to 114, or by 100 percent. In the succeeding period the index for medical price inflation slowed considerably.

Another factor should be borne in mind. From 1985 to 1994, the population of New York City increased by a minimal 1 percent. Although the non-census year figures are, at best, projections that are compounded by the difficulties of reaching minority populations and more particularly, undocumented immigrants, the estimates of the New York City population for 1985 and 1994 used by the New York City Planning Commission are 7.2 million and 7.3 million respectively.

Another revealing index of national health care expenditures during the past two decades are the changes in the percentage of GDP contributed by health care. In 1985 the proportion of health care was 10.5 percent; the figure for 1994 is close to 14 percent, or an increase of just under 40 percent. In the preceding decade the percentage rose from 8.6 to 10.5, reflecting a much lower rate of increase.

Many market-oriented economists believe that the United States has entered an era of much constrained expenditures for health care services which they attribute to the rapid expansion of managed care plans with their focus on achieving economies, particularly through the reduced use of in-patient hospital care, by far the most costly of all health services. Although these optimistic conclusions that the annual increases in national health care spending are finally on a downward trend may turn out

TABLE 3.2

Projected Personal Health Care Expenditures by Major Component: 1995

Component	Amount ($ billion)
Hospitals	365
Nursing home and home care	circa 80
Physicians' services	200
	645
All other components including dentists' services, other professionals, drugs, net cost of insurance and administration	255
	$900 billion

Source: Burner, S.T. and Waldo, D.R. "National Health Care Projections, 1994–2005." *Health Care Financing Review*, Summer 1995.

to be correct, there is little in the nation's experience thus far that would justify such certainty.

Detailed projections of national health expenditures for the coming decade have been calculated by senior staff members of the Office of the Actuary and the U.S. Health Care Financing Administration and this is how the estimated figures look for the end of 1994:

The figures for the decade 1985 to 1995 indicate that personal health care spending in the U.S. rose from $380.5 billion to $900 billion for a total increase of 137 percent, a rate slightly greater than those for the two preceding decades. The fact that there was no deceleration in the rate of increase despite strenuous efforts by the federal government to moderate its outlays by the introduction of a prospective system of hospital reimbursement in 1984, subsequent efforts to slow the rate of payments to physicians treating Medicare patients, and the reduced rate of increase in the medical price index during the past decade is a potent reminder of the ability of the health care system to continue to extract additional funds from the rest of the economy. The financial flows into the health care sector are not likely to be significantly altered unless the health care sector and/or the economy at large come(s) face to face with major disequilibrating forces.

In the case of New York City we do not have a set of accounts that provides us with sound comprehensive information for the third decade, 1986 to 1994, and must therefore make use of estimates.

The UHF study estimated total personal health care expenditures of New York City in 1985 to be just under $17 billion. Our estimate for 1994 is $44 billion which represents an increase of 159 percent, about 16 percent higher than the U.S. as a whole where outlays rose by 137 percent.

As a reasonable first approximation, using $44 billion as the total New York City expenditure for health care in 1994, the three principal components—hospitals, $21 billion; physician services, $9.7 billion; and nursing home and home care, $3.8 billion—accounted for about 78 percent, substantially the same as a decade earlier.

Within these parameters significant changes were occurring, specifically, a decline in hospital admissions and a modest parallel decline in the average length of stay. However, ambulatory care increased. As for long-term care, New York City experienced a very large increase in home care expenditures reported by the New York State Department of Social Services to be over $1.4 billion in 1994.

The relative shares of public and private spending for health care continued to be 54 percent and 46 percent respectively.

As we shall see in the next chapter, the health care system in New York City faced a number of acute challenges as well as some opportunities during the last decade. The striking fact that emerges, however, is the continuing strong upward surge in total spending. In commenting on "The Changing Health Care Environment" in December 1994, the Governor's Health Care Advisory Board observed that, "The overall growth in New York State's health care expenditures parallels national trends and represents a thirty-year pattern of increases at about three times the general inflation rate." This statement regarding New York State applies as well to New York City. A veritable cascade of additional funds flowed in from the four principal funding sources led by private health insurance and Medicaid which accounted for two-thirds; Medicare and out-of-pocket payments together with "other" constituted the remaining third.

During the three decades between 1965 and 1994 personal health care expenditures in constant dollars doubled in New York City although the population declined from about 8 million to about 7 million in 1975 and is now estimated at 7.3 million.

The following summary table shows the rise (in current and constant dollars) in total expenditures for personal health care services in New York City for each of the three decades.

TABLE 3.3

Expenditures for Personal Health Care Services in New York City: 1965, 1976, 1985, 1994

	Current $	Constant $*	Percent change in Constant $
1965	$2.5 bil	$9.9 bil	
1976	8.3	16	62
1985	17.0	15	(–6)
1994	44.0	20	33
			Cumulative 102

*1982–84=100

Sources: 1965, 1976 Piore
1985, 1994 UHF

The rate of national personal health expenditures (in constant dollars) over the same period, rose considerably faster than that of New York City. However, the nation's population grew by about a third during these three decades while the New York City population declined about 8 percent. With these adjustments, the difference is largely obliterated. The increase in spending in constant dollars comes to about 110 percent for the U.S. and 125 percent for New York City.

This brings us to the nub of the matter: although the number of dollars flowing into the health care system in New York has increased substantially, there is little evidence of commensurate improvements in the health care of the poor. A cursory look at epidemiological and demographic data for the period reveals that while health indices for the poor have improved in absolute terms, the differential between the poor and the nonpoor remains the same. Perhaps reflecting the above, the relative measures of health status for whites and nonwhites have not changed. There is an almost two-to-one difference in infant mortality rates, even as the rates for both groups have been declining.

If the dollars did not directly improve health status, what have they done? Clearly, one impact of the increased spending on the poor has been to raise the wages of health workers and physicians and to improve the capital position of hospitals and health facilities. Moreover, the number of people employed in the health system has increased substantially. The health sector went from being the seventh largest employer in New York City in 1960 to the third largest in 1970, with a current workforce of above 300,000. As other industries have waxed and waned, health employment has increased steadily through major recessions and economic droughts. Not only have large numbers of city residents been employed in the health sector, their wages and salaries have increased as well. The ability of the institutional workers in the health sector to obtain higher wages has traditionally been linked to the use of public sector funds to increase wages. The introduction of Medicare and Medicaid served to intensify this process since the lion's share of the new money came directly from the federal government.

An additional factor that must be considered in understanding the impact of the new flow of dollars into the health field is that many of the newly employed personnel in the health sector were recent immigrants or native born minorities. Between 1975 and 1995 the number employed in the health services industry in New York City increased from 185,000 to 295,000 or by 60 percent. In many cases, the jobs required little, if any, skill or experience and accordingly enabled individuals who might otherwise have been on welfare to be self-supporting. In assessing the impact of massive health care spending, this untargetted but critical gain should not be underestimated.

4

The Role of the State

New York State indisputably has the most highly regulated health care system in the nation. It was the first state to legislate a certificate of need program; it has regulated hospital reimbursement rates for almost fifteen years, and it has long maintained a system of subsidizing uncompensated hospital care that serves to ensure access to in-patient services for those unable to pay their bills. A major focus of these regulations has been the need to provide for those in poverty, the vast majority of whom live in New York City. In addition to the city's public hospital system and public health programs, these state initiatives have served as the principal vehicles for providing essential health care to the poor in New York, and as such deserve particular attention.

Since the 1930s, New York City has maintained a capital system for its public hospitals. In 1966 the state inaugurated its own certificate of need law that went far beyond the stipulations of the Comprehensive Health Planning Act which was enacted by Congress that year. For New York City, health planning meant that efforts to expand existing hospitals or establish new ones required certificates of operation that obligated them to maintain emergency rooms and to provide charity care. Along with the large number of public hospitals that were owned and operated by the city, these provisions expanded access for the poor to basic hospital services.

The concentration of teaching hospitals in New York City has also played an important role in the care of the poor. Teaching hospitals have always had need to attract and treat poor patients in order to perform their teaching functions. While much of the care of the poor devolved onto hospital housestaff and medical students, and often engendered community-hospital tensions, the arrangement served the needs of both groups reasonably well. The quid pro quo was further institutionalized with the initiation of affiliation agreements between municipal hospitals and major medical schools/teaching hospitals beginning in the early 1960s.

The immediate impetus for this policy was the imminent disaccreditation in 1961 of Harlem Hospital because of the poor quality of care rendered to patients. An agreement was struck by the New York City commissioner of hospitals with Columbia University to provide professional staffing for the hospital. This initial one million dollar plus agreement has since evolved into a $500 million (as of 1995) program that covers nine of the eleven acute care facilities of the Health and Hospitals Corporation (two have arrangements with professional corporations that are not affiliated with medical schools or hospitals). The affiliation of the municipal hospitals with medical schools and teaching hospitals allowed for the easier integration of teaching and research with patient care for a patient population that was implicitly poor. The improvement of the quality of the municipal hospitals through the 1960s and early 1970s was clearly an outcome of this affiliation policy, reinforced by the flow of new dollars.

The passage of the New York Prospective Hospital Reimbursement Methodology (NYPHRM) in 1982 was a milestone for New York State as it attempted to address several pressing problems related to the provision of hospital services. Since the system stipulated permissible levels of cost shifting between third parties (e.g., commercial insurance rates were 13 percent higher than Blue Cross or Medicaid), and hospitals had no other sources of income, there had to be a mechanism to deal with uncompensated care. As conventionally defined, uncompensated hospital care consists of charity care (care knowingly rendered free or below cost) and bad debt (services for which reimbursement is expected but not received). To deal with these issues, NYPHRM established a series of eight regional pools in New York State. Hospitals in each region were required to pay a surcharge of approximately 5 percent (1995) of their non-Medicare gross revenues into this pool and the money would be redistributed based on the amount of bad debt and charity care that each hospital in the region generated. The purpose of the regional pools was to limit the political liability of shifting money from upstate New York to New York City where most of the uncompensated care was provided. Beyond this simple redistributive mechanism, there was an additional scheme which allowed hospitals that were declared to be fiscally distressed to recover 100 percent of their bad debt and charity care before the remaining hospitals in the region could draw on what was left in the pool. This second mechanism had the effect of ensuring the survival of hospitals in the poorest neighborhoods where health insurance coverage was lowest. However, this approach has proved to be a precarious mechanism since the nondistressed hospitals receive less and less money and are therefore liable to drift into "distress." This has in fact been the case in New York City where a number of the larger hospitals sink into a progressively deeper financial morass as a smaller percentage of their uncompensated care is returned to them. In 1995 over $1 billion in bad debt and charity care was redistributed in New York via this mechanism. In addition to the bad debt and charity care pools, $6.5 billion in hospital care was paid for by Medicaid and another $300 million of city tax levy funds was received by municipal (HHC) hospitals.

The New York City Health and Hospitals Corporation is the largest municipal system in the United States with, as noted above, eleven acute care hospitals containing 7,000 beds, two chronic care hospitals, four nursing homes, an HMO (Metro-Plus) and a large number of ambulatory clinics. No other city or county provides this range and volume of health care services to its poor and uninsured residents, though New York City may be forced to reduce the level of service provision in the near future. The former Department of Hospitals of the city was administratively responsible at one time for seventeen hospitals in what was clearly an inefficient and ineffective system. There was no centralization in planning, equipment, or quality control; staffing was limited by city civil service titles and salaries; and purchasing was done through the central city purchasing department. The changes in financing brought about by the enactment of Medicare and Medicaid, the quality problems that necessitated academic affiliation agreements, and the desire to improve the delivery of services led to the exploration of new models of public medical services delivery. These considerations resulted in the creation in 1971 of the Health and Hospitals Corporation (HHC), established as a quasi-public agency with an independent board of directors (although the majority of appointees to the board are made by the mayor). The HHC was free of civil service titles and salaries and could do its own purchasing. It could also issue its own debt. The general agreement was that the city would make up the deficit of the HHC from tax levy funds up to a predetermined level.

The HHC was created so that nonpublic hospitals could become part of the Corporation, but this never happened. The HHC began to run into problems as soon as it was established. One of the precipitants reflected the unionization of health care workers. A large number of voluntary hospitals in New York were organized, principally by the National Health and Human Services Workers Union, Local 1199, an offshoot of the older pharmacists' union. Municipal hospitals were organized by District Council 37 of the American Federation of State, County, and Municipal Employees (AFSCME). The bifurcated unionization structure made it difficult to explore the potential for encompassing the voluntary hospitals in the HHC or converting public hospitals into private institutions. The New York City fiscal crisis, which reached its zenith in 1975, also became a factor as the HHC found it difficult to raise capital, and annual subsidies from the city began to decline resulting in severe budgetary pressure on the public hospitals. Perhaps the most serious problem was rapid turnover of senior management at the HHC. Presidents tended to last less than a year either because of frustration with the job, lack of competence, conflict with City Hall, turnover of the mayoralty, and substantially higher compensation in the private sector. The problems that affected the central administration also affected the management of the individual hospitals.

The individual hospitals had always been hotbeds of political patronage which the new centralized system was designed to minimize and eliminate. This did not happen. Administrators were loath to make technological improvements that would lead to a smaller workforce, nor were they anxious to antagonize the political forces that could have an impact on their own tenure.

While HHC was suffering through these birth and growing pains, the voluntary hospitals were prospering through the financial benefits of Medicaid and Medicare and had embarked on modernization campaigns. As municipal hospitals grew older (and obsolescent), voluntary hospitals were rejuvenated. The result was that private patients (i.e., patients with private health insurance) rarely used public hospitals. Even the elderly poor who had been dependent on the public system prior to Medicare, now found themselves admitted to private hospitals by their private physicians. The public system filled up with Medicaid patients and the uninsured, and this further served to keep privately insured patients away.

By the mid- to late 1980s, the HHC began to confront its identity as a provider of care to the poor. Its mission statement was changed to reflect this newly perceived self-image, and it broadened its scope of care for the poor beyond acute care hospitalization and outpatient and emergency services. The HHC began to plot a strategy to provide improved primary care services to its patient population. This entailed the development of new primary care centers, the conversion of older, disease-specific clinics to primary care centers, and the reorganization of outpatient departments into primary care units.

Yet it soon became clear that while the HHC wished to provide poor people with improved access to primary care, many didn't necessarily want what was offered. Patients learned that receipt of an appointment card with a specified time and date did not eliminate the need to wait in an uncomfortable room for several hours before being seen. They also learned that having an ongoing relationship with a particular physician was exceeedingly difficult in the face of high staff turnover. They learned that even with a fair degree of computerization, records could rarely be found and patients either received the same diagnostic services repeatedly or never received them at all.

Health management experts recognized that these problems were a reflection of the difficulty of running a 50,000-person health care organization, with restricted financial resources, and the inherent bureaucracy of political organizations. Clearly, with more time, more money, and better managerial talent, the HHC might become an effective provider of primary care services—but to date the time and money and talent have not been forthcoming. Nevertheless, despite these problems, the sheer volume of care that HHC provides to its client population is truly impressive.

The other major public provider of health care for the poor has been the New York City Department of Health (DOH). New York City had established one of the first health departments in the country which became the model for similar departments in other cities and states. Its direct health care services included well- and sick baby clinics, sexually transmitted disease (STD) and later AIDS clinics, tuberculosis and infectious disease clinics, school health clinics, dental clinics, and many others. These clinics were located in low-income communities and many—most—had a good reputation for service provision. The decline of the DOH system began after the onset of the city's fiscal crisis in 1975 when the budget of the department was cut by almost 50 percent and an administrative decision was made to terminate the direct provision and delivery of services by the Department in favor of the expanded regulation and monitoring of health care services.

The impact of this decision did not become apparent for several years since the overall budget and staffing cuts so decimated the Department that the specific effects of this policy change could not be readily evaluated. In practice, when the clinics closed, people either went to other clinics and waited longer to obtain service, or they went to public and voluntary hospital outpatient departments for care. While city officials contended that poor people were not losing access to essential services since they could still use the OPDs, the range and quality of care they received was seldom evaluated.

The DOH clinics were organized to provide preventive services and a substantial component of health education was included as part of each patient's visit. Patients who were acutely ill were referred to a medical facility. Since the hospital OPDs did not aim to provide preventive services, patients who came with any health complaint whatever were treated as requiring acute care. No health education was provided. The net result of this change was that less preventive care was provided and many who utilized these services tended to wait until they were acutely ill before seeking medical attention. Even after the HHC made its commitment to primary care in the latter 1980s, the clinics that it operated tended to utilize a medical rather than a preventive model of care. This, in retrospect, seems to have been a serious policy error.

Perhaps the most important preventive services mediated by the Department of Health were those provided through the school health program. New York City established the first school health program in the nation and it achieved such a high level of effectiveness that when the state introduced regulations governing the operation of school health programs in other areas, the city was exempted because its standards were so much higher.

In general, all school children were required to have a certificate attesting to a medical examination and a dental examination in the preceding six months in order to register for school. Those students who could not afford private medical care could obtain the required services at a health department clinic. In addition, each class was screened at least once a year for vision and hearing problems.

With the fiscal crisis of the mid-1970s, the school health program was cut back substantially. It was relatively easy to do this since the city was exempt from state guidelines in this arena. Not only was routine screening cut back, but the number of school nurses was severely reduced. By the early 1990s, there were fewer than one nurse for every 14,000 students—a ratio that, for all intents and purposes, is tantamount to having no school health program at all. It should also be noted that since it is no longer possible for the DOH to guarantee medical and dental visits, this component of the program has been suspended as well. A 1989 Mayor's Commission on the Future of Child Health in New York City revealed that it took well over a year between the time a child was screened for visual or aural deficiency and the actual remediation of the problem.

Further, school health programs have focused more on mental health/sex education/social services for early teens and adolescents than on the health needs of preteens and elementary school students. This has led the school health program to become embroiled in public controversies over the proper auspices and site for sex education, the teaching of abstinence, teenage pregnancy prevention, condom distribution, and AIDS education.

The final major source of health care for the poor in New York City has been the various community health centers that have been established since the mid-1960s. The first wave of clinics originated with federal funds via the Office of Economic Opportunity and tended to be very large, comprehensive ambulatory care centers. A second wave of clinics came through the Urban Health Initiative program (Section 330) and these tended to be more like storefront clinics with two or three physicians per site. The final wave of clinics consists of former Department of Health clinics that have been transferred to the Health and Hospitals Corporation. In addition, the city, in 1991 enacted the Communicare Program—with the objective of transforming categorical or disease-specific clinics into primary care centers. The plans call for the opening of sixty such clinics in New York City. Supplementing these community clinic efforts has been the establishment of the Primary Care Development Corporation (PCDC), which is designed to provide capital to clinics and hospitals that wish to expand their primary care capacity. Prior to the establishment of PCDC, it was extremely difficult for new ambulatory care centers to obtain capital support. The sponsorship of the successor Communicare II clinics is no longer limited to HHC but includes nonprofit community agencies.

In all, the existing clinics provide over 1,000,000 ambulatory visits annually and although this amounts to less than 10 percent of the total ER and OPD visits provided by hospitals in New York City, it is nevertheless a significant figure.

New York City has the highest physician to population ratio of any major U.S. urban area. Yet, physicians in private practice are not a major source of medical care for the poor. It is estimated that less than 15 percent of all physicians participate in the Medicaid program, and most do so in institutional settings rather than in their private practices. New York City contains a large number of Medicaid Mills—high-volume clinics catering to Medicaid beneficiaries—but numerous studies have found that they offer little preventive care, do not do a good job in providing routine services, and send all complicated cases to emergency rooms. A major percentage of the Medicaid Mill doctors are international medical graduates who as a rule do not have hospital admitting privileges. A growing number of native practitioners and traditional healers have also settled in New York, largely in immigrant communities. These range from acupuncturists in Chinatown to herbal physicians in the Dominican community of Washington Heights, to emigré Soviet physicians who are not licensed to practice in the U.S. While there is no reliable count of the number of such physicians practicing in New York City and the volume of care they provide, it appears from anecdotal evidence that the supply continues to grow.

The assumption is that Medicaid managed care will be a spur to the expanded provision of primary care by private practitioners, but thus far this has not happened to any significant degree. Most of the new managed care companies contract with established clinics or build new clinics so that physicians do not have to see Medicaid patients in their private offices.

There are several related developments that have stimulated efforts to provide improved health care to the poor. These include state insurance reforms, primary care initiatives, and capital funding for distressed hospitals.

The dominant provider of health insurance in New York has been Empire Blue Cross Blue Shield. In recognition of its role as insurer of last resort, the company was allowed a discount of 13 percent from the standard hospital insurance rate. Even with this discount, the company claimed to be losing money on its individual and small group contracts. In response, the legislature enacted insurance reform legislation in 1993 requiring all insurance companies doing business in the state to offer insurance policies to individuals (i.e., nongroup coverage) or else pay an extra surcharge on their hospital rates which would go to Blue Cross.

Further, the legislature required that all insurers use a single "community" rate in pricing their insurance for a series of demographically defined groups. The aim of this legislation was to permit insurance costs for individuals not eligible for group policies to be reduced. The early results of this policy indicate that an increased number of insurance firms are selling individual policies, but they also show that while premiums for some high use groups have been reduced, premiums for the entire community have risen. This finding was used during the debates on national health legislation in 1994 as an argument against community rating in the potential reform of health insurance.

A second state action related to insurance coverage was the introduction of Child Health Plus, an ambulatory care insurance program for children with costs ranging from zero to a sliding scale fee based on total family income. The program was developed by the late commissioner of health, David Axelrod, whose vision inspired most of the developments in New York State from the late 1970s to the early 1990s that had an impact on the health of the poor. The program was designed for families not eligible for Medicaid, but for whom private health insurance was not a viable option. It was funded through a diversion of funds from the bad debt and charity care pools based on the premise that if people had insurance, they would not generate so much uncompensated care. The hospitals resisted this diversion of funds from the pool, and although unsuccessful in blocking the new program, they were able to limit the amount of money that went into it and hence limit the number of families that could participate. Over 100,000 families are currently enrolled in the program.

It should also be noted that New York State has taken advantage of federal mandates to increase the eligibility ceiling for women and children on Medicaid to the maximum allowed level. At present this covers women and newborns up to 185 percent of the poverty level, those with children aged one to six up to 133 percent of the poverty level, and those with children aged seven to twelve up to 100 percent. This expansion was financed 50 percent by the federal government, 25 percent by the state government and 25 percent by local counties (including New York City).

New York State has also used monies from the bad debt and charity care pools to fund a variety of primary care initiatives—projects and demonstrations designed to increase the numbers and types of primary care providers and also to expand the facilities' capacity for primary care.

One of the most controversial programs developed by New York State was the fiscally distressed hospitals capital fund. Hospitals serving inner-city areas in which many of the patients are not insured, are as a rule not in good financial shape and generally have great difficulty gaining access to the capital markets. What prudent investor would lend money to a hospital that stood a good chance of going out of business well before its debt could be repaid? Hospitals serving the poor in New York were in even further jeopardy since the rate regulation system prohibited them from cost-shifting and thus compensating for losses from charity and bad debt cases with revenues from better insured patients.

Given this situation, New York State passed legislation that enabled fiscally distressed institutions to access a pool of money raised via New York State's credit rating. The hospitals are required to establish depreciation funds and to submit to fiscal monitoring by the New York Medical Care Facilities Financing Authority (MCFFA). At present, eleven hospitals have been designated as fiscally distressed by the Department of Health; seven are located in New York City (Bronx-Lebanon, North General, Interfaith, Wyckoff Heights, Jamaica, St. Clare's, Brookdale). As of mid-1995, four have received an average of $150 million each to rebuild their capital plants.

What seemed like a novel and progressive idea when it was proposed in the late 1980s, must now be viewed in a different light. With the state DOH projecting that over 20 percent of New York State's acute care capacity is surplus and expecting hospitals to be downsized and closed over the next few years, the wisdom of building new facilities for a population that cannot generally afford hospital care and that must be kept operational so as not to cause a default which the state would be obligated to cover looks in retrospect to have been more problematic.

It should be noted that it is not easy for any hospital in New York to obtain access to the capital markets. The fiscally distressed program assists only those hospitals that the state has declared to be in distress, a judgment that does not imply that other hospitals are necessarily in sound financial shape. Moreover, the program applies only to voluntary hospitals. Even large academic centers in New York require help in securing capital to rebuild or expand. The major source of this funding has been the Federal Housing Authority hospital mortgage program (section 242), a mortgage insurance program. New York City hospitals comprise 86 percent of the entire portfolio of the FHA program. Over the past decade virtually all the major medical centers in New York City have undergone either total renovation or substantial modernization. The average cost of these projects has been in the $500–$600 million range. The New York Hospital is currently embarked on a $600 million program to upgrade its plant. These capital expenditures which have increased the costs of hospital care in the city were necessitated, so the hospitals argue, by their need to remain up to date and competitive with other facilities both in the city and around the world. However, as the occupancy rates and lengths of stay drop these presumptions and decisions must be reassessed. The possibility of hospital default is real. The recent cutback in Medicaid spending in New York and the forthcoming federal Medicare and Medicaid cuts have made the FHA extremely wary about its investment in New York hospitals.

The Health and Hospitals Corporation has the authority to issue its own debt but internal problems have blocked the implementation of needed upgrading projects. Kings County Hospital is a case in point. Kings County is a complex of 26 buildings in the Flatbush section of Brooklyn. It is the largest hospital in the borough and the primary teaching hospital of the State University of New York College of Medicine at Brooklyn (SUNY Downstate), located across the street. Plans to rebuild the facility, which is antiquated and extremely inefficient, have existed for decades, but in the late 1980s they began to take firm shape as a billion dollar project which would construct four new buildings—an acute care facility, a skilled nursing facility, a prison facility, and a mental health facility. Work was started on preliminary demolition and more detailed planning, but was derailed by exposés of rigged contracting and political favoritism. After more than $116 million had been spent, the HHC halted the project. It is unlikely that the project will be reactivated in the near future, as it will be difficult to raise the capital, Mayor Giuliani is not in favor of the project, and the need for a $1 billion dollar facility seems increasingly remote at this time of declining hospital utilization. Plans for the renovation of other HHC facilities have similarly been put on hold.

In summary, New York provides an extraordinary amount of health services to its poor. The commitment of public as well as private resources to the care of the poor has been long standing and deep, and although the financial position of many of the institutions that deliver care has changed, the commitment remains. The hospitals in New York were not major advocates of universal health care, at least in the form presented in President Clinton's health reform proposals of 1993 and 1994. Since the hospitals in New York City had long provided the equivalent of universal care to the city's residents, their major concern was to maintain their financial viability, something that might be jeopardized if the reforms were enacted. The reforms contemplated the reorganization and financing of graduate medical education in ways that would not have been helpful to New York City, surely not in the short run. Moreover, the reforms threatened hospital revenues by reducing if not eliminating such sources as disproportionate share payments from Medicare and Medicaid. The hospitals in New York City were also concerned about the strong commitment of the reforms to the rapid growth of managed care.

Yet, as we look ahead to the end of this century and beyond, many or most of these issues may turn out to be moot. The hospitals in New York City are busy forming new alliances and systems to meet the many challenges that loom ahead including but not limited to the further growth of managed care. They may decide in retrospect, that their earlier cautionary stance towards national health care reform was not an optimal strategy.

5

How Much Did Health Care
for the Poor Improve?

A good place to begin this chapter is to inquire how well the poor in New York City fared in obtaining medical care at the time that the nation took a major step forward in passing Medicare and Medicaid. We have noted earlier the city's long tradition of providing access to health care for all New Yorkers, irrespective of ability to pay, principally in its municipal hospitals and clinics. In the early 1960s, however, the acute shortfall in physician personnel at the municipal hospitals meant that most of the poor received seriously substandard ambulatory and inpatient care.

Smaller numbers of the poor continued to receive care in the clinics and inpatient services of hospitals under voluntary auspices, especially the leading teaching hospitals that played key roles at the frontiers of medical education, research, and patient care. However, with their own budgets seldom yielding a surplus, most voluntary hospitals had to curtail the amount of free and below cost care that they were able and willing to provide the poor.

There are several different perspectives from which to explore the issue of whether and to what extent access of the poor to essential health care services in New York City improved over the last three decades. The first is to compare quantitatively the essential health care services available to the poor in 1995 as opposed to 1965. A second would be to examine the differences in access to and quality of health care between the poor and the nonpoor at the start and end of the thirty-year period. Still another approach would be to take account of the gains in medical knowledge and technique over the period and assess how well the poor fared in light of the health system's growing capabilities. Presumably, one could formulate other criteria by which to measure advances in the health care for the poor during these years, but these seem fundamental.

47

As we emphasized in chapter 2, ours is a highly pluralistic health care financing and delivery system so that any inquiry into the altered circumstances of one of the key parties must also look into other key parties, specifically physicians, hospitals, health care workers and their trade unions, insurers, and the several levels of government all of which are primarily engaged in pursuing their own interests and goals even while they are involved in providing and improving care to the city's poor.

It is well to remember that national health reform in 1965 was targeted at the elderly—the vast majority of whom at the time were poor or within 200 percent of the poverty standard—and had no assured access to mainstream medical care once they retired. Medicare was designed as a social insurance mechanism whose purpose was to make certain that the nation's working population would have access on retirement to mainstream health care services (defined as treatment by fee-for-service physicians of their own choosing and acute care hospitalization in voluntary as well as public hospitals for inpatient diagnostic and therapeutic services when needed).

Medicare was not an open-ended entitlement. It required the elderly to cover co-payments and deductibles; it did not include long-term care benefits either for routine nursing home care or home care; and it did not cover drugs and, most important, preventive services. However in the years and decades that followed, the federal government introduced important changes that contributed to the well-being of the elderly. It stipulated in 1972 that their Social Security benefits would be indexed to changes in the cost of living; it amended Medicaid so that those who met its eligibility criteria, including the elderly, could be admitted for routine nursing home care; in 1989 when most of the 1988 Catastrophic Amendments to Medicare were revoked, Medicaid was mandated to pay the costs of deductibles and co-payments for Medicare enrollees whose incomes were below the poverty level, and it introduced other revisions in Medicare rules and regulations that enabled the elderly to utilize more fully mainstream medical care.

The favorable impact of Medicare on the New York City elderly was reflected in the fact that soon after implementation of the new statute, the large elderly poor population who had previously obtained much of their care from the municipal hospital sector had found their way to the private offices of fee-for-service practitioners and to voluntary hospitals.

Another way of summarizing the changed circumstances of the pre-Medicare poor and near poor elderly population is to note that the federal government, with periodic assists from the federal-state Medicaid programs, fulfilled its commitment to enable the elderly to obtain care from the mainstream health care delivery system. It further contributed directly to improving their economic circumstances by indexing Social Security benefits to the cost of living which helped to reduce the proportion of the poor among the elderly from about one in three to about one in ten.

Although in 1995 most of the elderly are no longer poor or particularly handicapped in obtaining mainstream medical care, this is not true for all. According to the New York State Department of Social Services, the 2 million Medicaid-eligible individuals in New York City in late 1994 included just under 200,000 older persons—125,000 recipients of supplementary security income (SSI) from the federal government and another 71,000 who received no income support but were eligible for medical assistance.

During the third quarter of 1994, about 152,000 SSI and medical assistance recipients incurred some 900 million dollars of health care expenditures out of a total outlay for the city of just under $3 billion. Half of the expenditures for the SSI-aged went for personal care and home health services; the other large outlay categories were hospitalization and nursing home care. In the case of the aged who received medical assistance only, 70 percent of the $567 million expenditures for this category went for nursing home care. What these figures indicate is that the elderly in New York City who required special government assistance to meet their medical expenses in 1994 were for the most part those in need of services that are not adequately covered by Medicare, that is, nursing home care and home care. An alternative formulation is that between 1966 and 1995 the federal government, largely through its own initiatives to provide income support and medical services for the elderly, went most of the way to relieve this population of the twin threats of poverty and inadequate access to mainstream medical care.

The poor in New York City and elsewhere have never consisted predominantly of the elderly. Most of the poor are children and adults receiving benefits from the Aid to Families with Dependent Children program (AFDC); the rest are adults and related children on home relief, a category that is not funded by the federal government. Of the 2 million Medicaid eligibles in New York City in September 1994, 886,000 (278,000 adults and 608,000 children) were AFDC recipients. Another 287,000 (234,000 adults and 53,000 children) were home relief clients.

In short, the AFDC and home relief populations accounted for about 59 percent of all Medicaid eligibles.

But this is not the whole story. Though recipients of AFDC and home relief represent over half of all Medicaid eligibles, only 16 percent of total Medicaid outlays were spent on their behalf. To account for the balance of Medicaid beneficiaries and expenditures, we must add the category of the blind and disabled.

During the period we are examining they numbered 190,000 (17 percent) of the 1.1 million monthly average of individuals receiving medical services. However, just under half of all expenditures were made on their behalf. It is commonly perceived that Medicaid and other forms of public assistance for health care go overwhelmingly to adults and children on welfare—AFDC and home relief—but the above figures indicate clearly that in New York City it is the aged, the blind, and the disabled who are the principal beneficiaries of medical assistance.

The first and surely the most unequivocal fact summarizing the course of the last three decades is the vast increase in public expenditures for health care services to the residents of New York City and the American people at large. The outlays for Medicare and Medicaid have been focused respectively on the elderly and the poor, in particular the blind and the disabled. In New York City public dollars currently comprise slightly more than half of the $44 billion expended for health care as contrasted with 29 percent in 1965.

Another facet of the summary must be an assessment of the improvements in the health care services that the New York City poor (and elderly) obtained as a consequence of this large-scale inflow of public dollars. Here it is necessary to differentiate between the elderly and the poor who are entitled to a wide range of governmentally financed health care services and the uninsured who lack any form of coverage, public or private. A rough estimate of the number of uninsured persons in New York City, taking into consideration the large group of undocumented aliens, approximates 1.5 million. One must recall, however, that even the uninsured in New York City are entitled to medical care once they appear at one of the HHC hospitals or clinics for treatment. The question that we must confront is, how do the health care services available to the New York City elderly and poor in 1995 compare to those available to them in 1965?

In brief reply: The elderly are much better off because Medicare has provided them for the most part with access to mainstream medical care.

Further, in the intervening decades the health care financing and delivery systems have been broadened so that public dollars now finance long-term nursing home and home care services, although the elderly and the poor must qualify for Medicaid in order to gain access to these important services. Public dollars have also gone a considerable distance to enable both the voluntary and public hospitals, clinics, and diagnostic and treatment centers to undertake new interventions and procedures. Many patients who would have died in 1965 leave the hospital in good condition in 1995.

The foregoing is the positive side of the assessment. There is a downside as well. The large HHC infrastructure which is a principal and, for many of the poor, the sole provider of health care has confronted serious problems throughout the three decades in obtaining the range of resources that it requires to provide timely and efficient care to its large constituency—adequate numbers of competent physicians; nurse and support personnel; management and system capabilities; capital funding for maintenance, new construction, and costly new technology. In the presence of such severe resource constraints, the poor who seek treatment in these institutions are at a disadvantage in obtaining appropriate and timely care.

Some of the more serious shortfalls in the health care experience of many of the city's poor result from faults in the organization, management, staffing, and facilities of the HHC hospitals and clinics. The long waiting times for an initial clinic appointment or for treatment in the emergency room have been a source of continuing complaint on the part of poor patients who have little or no option but to make use of HHC facilities. The fact that many of the residents—in fact, the overwhelming majority—are international medical graduates (IMGs), often from non-English speaking countries, makes for poor communication between physician and patient. Since the patient's prior medical record, even for treatment in the same institution, can seldom be retrieved immediately, the physician on call must proceed with no guidance from the patient's medical history.

The Report of the Mayoral Commission to Review the Health and Hospitals Corporation (Barondess Commission) appointed in 1992 by Mayor David Dinkins found serious deficiencies on the part of many of the affiliated AHCs in the supervision of their residents who were placed in one or another of the HHC institutions. Because of the shortcomings identified in the municipal hospitals, the residency review committees (RRCs) and other accrediting agencies have repeatedly cited the weaker HHC hospitals and on occasion suspended or terminated one or another residency training program.

Nevertheless, most poor New Yorkers who seek treatment at an HHC institution obtain satisfactory care even if it is oriented primarily to the treatment of acute, episodic illness rather than the provision of a comprehensive range of preventive, primary care, acute care and follow-up services that would contribute more effectively to maintaining the health of the individual and the family over the long term.

We now need to shift focus and consider briefly how the city's poor have fared in terms of access to neighborhood physicians in private practice; ambulatory and inpatient care at voluntary hospitals; and long-term care services in nursing homes and at home. To begin with, one must call attention to the fact that most voluntary hospitals distinguish between the poor who are eligible for Medicaid and those with no insurance coverage most of whom would find it difficult or impossible to pay for an ambulatory care visit. The latter are usually encouraged to seek treatment at an HHC hospital, especially if one is located close by.

Failing a true emergency, care in the emergency room of a voluntary hospital is likely to result in a less than optimal encounter for the poor just as it is in an HHC institution. The treating physician is seldom adequately informed about the patient's health status and prior medical history and the isolated encounter is often marked by poor communication and poor patient compliance.

Over the past several decades there have been notable gains for Medicaid-eligible persons in obtaining care in nursing homes or in home care programs. The latter was so successful that in the late 1980s the state of New York found it necessary for financial reasons to cap its contributions for the further expansion of Medicaid home care. Currently (mid-1995) the New York City Human Resources Administration has a total Medicaid home care caseload of 51,000.

There are various groups of poor persons, such as the homeless, individuals who live in shelters, the mentally ill, patients in an advanced stage of AIDS, drug addicts, individuals with active tuberculosis, and others afflicted with chronic health conditions whose socially dysfunctional behavior makes it very difficult for them to access and use the health care system effectively. Admittedly, such groups have always been part of the fabric of major metropolitan centers and they have always had difficulty in dealing with the societal support systems—including the health system; the fact remains, however, that the members of these groups receive less health care than they need or could use.

Still another, much larger group of the city's poor consists of persons with chronic conditions who are not effectively linked to the health care system in the sense that they must take the initiative in seeking ongoing medical attention. In turn, few of the health care providers—such as neighborhood hospitals, clinics, and others—have an effective outreach structure in place capable of following up patients after they have been initially treated.

How then do we answer the question of whether the health care of the poor improved? The elderly who became Medicare beneficiaries at age sixty-five realized the greatest gains because their enrollment in Medicare A and Medicare B, often supplemented by a privately purchased Medigap policy or Medicaid eligibility, assured most of them broad access to mainstream medical and nursing home or home care. The range and depth of the medical care now available to them far exceeds what it had been in 1965.

If we turn to the nonelderly poor, we find a less clear-cut set of outcomes. We will look first at the Medicaid eligible. While they have thus far had the option of being treated by private practitioners of their own choosing, in point of fact most low-income neighborhoods have long lacked an adequate supply of physicians able and willing to treat their residents at the prevailing Medicaid reimbursement rates. With few exceptions, only IMGs have tended to locate and practice in these neighborhoods. Although some of the poor who are eligible for Medicaid are able to obtain ambulatory care at neighborhood clinics and other essential community providers, for the most part they obtain their care at HHC and voluntary hospitals. When it comes to inpatient care, the majority of Medicaid patients are treated in voluntary hospitals, which on balance represents a gain over their pre-1965 situation.

The most vulnerable among the city's poor are the uninsured. Basically lacking any options about site of care, they must seek most of their medical care from HHC institutions. In the post-1965 era when the overwhelming majority of the city's population has been covered by either private or public health insurance, the uninsured have been the most marginal group.

In summary, most of the elderly poor enjoyed substantial gains by virtue of their ability to be treated by mainstream practitioners and specialists and to obtain inpatient treatment in voluntary hospitals, including the city's best. All of the city's poor gained access to long-term care in nursing homes or in home care programs which expanded greatly in the 1970s and 1980s. The uninsured poor—those who did not meet the eligibility criteria for Medicaid—were the most vulnerable and got the least. In the event of a serious illness requiring inpatient care they would most likely seek admission to an HHC hospital which, despite revenue and other constraints, was generally able to discharge most patients in a satisfactory condition.

One might ask, why explore what "others" got if our primary interest is in assessing the gains of the city's poor over the past three decades? Since the primary instrument for improving the health care of the nation's poor has been the large-scale new expenditures by the federal and state governments, why explore secondary and tertiary developments? The answer is simple and at the same time complex.

To begin with, the new funding that increased access to health care services for the elderly and the poor became the earnings and revenue streams for the providers of these services as well as for various intermediaries. And with more income at their command, the provider community was able to reassess its missions and goals. It is not only relevant but important to take note of some of the major gains that accrued to these secondary beneficiaries in New York City as a result of the new national health care policies.

We will start with physicians. Although they receive just one out of every five dollars of the total flow of health care expenditures, the decisions that they make play the key role in determining how most of the remaining medical care funds are distributed among the other major health care providers. The passage of Medicare and Medicaid and subsequent developments improved the earnings potential of physicians in New York City in several important ways. As we noted earlier, once the elderly were covered by Medicare they moved rapidly to seek out generalists and specialists whom earlier they could not afford to consult. Medicare assured the physicians who accepted them as patients of fees that were "customary, prevailing, and reasonable" for their area. This change was good for both parties—the physician community enlarged the number of paying patients in their private practices and a great many of the elderly were able to shift the locus of their care from the municipal system to mainstream fee-for-service.

Because of the low fee schedule set by the state of New York, the Medicaid-eligible population was for the most part unable to find private practitioners with a basic middle class clientele who were willing to accept them as private patients. However, Medicaid patients were generally welcomed as inpatients in the voluntary hospitals, including the AHCs, among other reasons because the respective heads of service were reimbursed at reasonable rates for their care and obtained additional reimbursement for supervising residents who performed most of the routine care that the Medicaid inpatients received.

The fact that Medicare and Medicaid reimbursed most physicians per unit of service that they provided enabled them to make use of more elaborate (and expensive) diagnostic and therapeutic interventions than they would have been inclined to use had the government not been picking up the bill. For instance, many physicians who practiced as members of a multispecialty or hospital-based group referred a significant proportion of their patients to one or more of their colleagues for evaluation and treatment, a practice that carried with it the promise of future reciprocity.

Given the Medicare population's free choice of physicians, it is not surprising to find that the last three decades have seen the rapid growth of specialists and subspecialists, particularly in New York City—long a center of sophisticated medicine—as more and more of the elderly, many of whom suffered from multiple chronic conditions, decided that they would do better under the care of a specialist.

In sum, the largely open-ended financing of physician services via Medicare's liberal reimbursement policies and the more restricted reimbursement for hospitalized Medicaid patients enabled the specialist community in New York City to maintain and improve its earnings in recent decades despite the steadily increasing number of physicians. While economics teaches us that increases in supply, other things being equal, tend to depress prices and earnings, other things were not equal in this case because of the ability of patients to choose the physicians whom they consulted; the broad discretion allowed physicians in selecting appropriate diagnostic and treatment modalities, and the obligation of third-party payers, primarily the federal and state governments, to pay the bills submitted.

Let us now consider how the new funding arrangements for Medicare and Medicaid affected the hospitals that provided all of the inpatient and much of the ambulatory care that the city's poor received. The voluntary hospitals, especially the large teaching hospitals, in New York City had always operated close to the margin: despite endowments and annual charitable contributions, their multiple missions usually exceeded their revenues. And the municipal hospitals were constrained by both lack of dollars and lack of physician personnel.

After the implementation of the new federal legislation, hospital revenues in New York City, particularly in the voluntary sector, improved dramatically as many hitherto charity and partial paying patients became, by virtue of Medicare and Medicaid, full-paying patients. Since Medicare reimbursed hospitals until 1983 on a cost-plus basis, the financial position of most voluntary institutions improved greatly inasmuch as third-party payers—private and public combined—covered over 90 percent of their total costs.

True, the state of New York continued to exercise tight control over many aspects of hospital operations via its certificate of need legislation requiring approval for all significant rebuilding or new construction; for the purchase of expensive technology or the introduction of new high cost procedures such as open heart surgery; and for the margins that the hospitals could strive to achieve. However, these restrictive rules and regulations should not obscure the fact that the post Medicare/Medicaid decades resulted in a significant improvement in the financial position of the city's voluntary hospitals.

The special funding that Medicare made available to hospitals with approved residency training programs (graduate medical education [GME]), the state-mandated contributions of other third-party payers for such training, and the disproportionate amount of GME performed under the auspices of the major teaching hospitals in New York City eventuated in a flow of $200,000 per resident per year (as of 1995) to the hospitals sponsoring approved residency programs.

Responding to the new sources of funding made available by Medicare and Medicaid, all of the AHCs in New York City—as in the rest of the country—enlarged their clinical staffs and offered faculty appointments to the new members. The practice plan revenue generated by these expanded clinical staffs became an important supplementary source of income to help support the combined missions of the AHCs—teaching, research, and patient care.

In the early 1980s the long-term upward trend in inpatient care started to level off but most hospitals were able to accommodate by expanding the scope of services that they provided on an ambulatory basis. And in the late 1980s-early 1990s, most New York City hospitals that provided large amounts of care to poor patients were able to obtain additional revenues from the "disproportionate share" payments that were reflected in the reimbursement formulas for both Medicare and Medicaid. Although the New York State regulatory authorities forced the hospitals in the state and in New York City to operate at conspicuously low net margins (less than 1 percent compared to over 4 percent for the nation as a whole since the early 1980s), Medicare and Medicaid helped to maintain a strong expansionary environment for the financing of voluntary hospitals. It should be noted that traditional measures of hospital operating efficiency such as margins and net revenue do not have the same significance in a highly regulated environment such as New York that they have elsewhere. Since uncompensated care is reimbursed, hospitals do not need comparable high margins to indicate fiscal soundness. Moreover, their ease in obtaining access to capital is in itself a reflection of the financial health of New York City hospitals, and obviates the need to maintain particularly high margins.

The situation was much more equivocal for the municipal hospitals. Between 1965 and 1975, with the benefit of additional funding from the new national programs, the HHC hospitals were enabled to improve the range and depth of their treatment programs. Subsequently, the city got caught up in a severe financial crisis in 1975 and remained immobilized until the early 1980s. To make matters worse, the HHC encountered great difficulties in modernizing its billing system to ensure that it received the payments due it; reforms were not fully implemented until the early 1980s. Only a year or two later, the HHC system was overwhelmed by the wave of new AIDS patients and other special patient groups for whom the city had primary responsibility. And at the end of the decade both the voluntary and municipal hospitals faced the double challenge of gridlocked beds and a severe shortage of registered nurses, a situation that fortunately turned out to be relatively short-lived.

A third party of interest that profited from Medicare and Medicaid funding were the many hospital employees that in the 1960s had begun to organize under the umbrella of two trade unions (Local 1199 for the voluntary hospitals, District Council 37 for the municipal hospitals) and gained considerable membership and strength in the 1970s. With cost-plus reimbursement, the administrators of the voluntary hospitals became less hostile than they had been to collective bargaining and gradually acceded to many union demands. When a stalemate threatened, the negotiating team was broadened informally to include the governor in Albany and the mayor in New York City each of whom had long-term political alliances with the unions and were therefore able to effect acceptable settlements by promising the hospitals that their increased wage and benefit costs would be reflected in their new reimbursement rates. In subsequent years, as reimbursement controls tightened via NYPHRM, the state of New York provided extra funding for issues of special interest and concern to the trade unions, such as assistance to displaced workers and money for training programs that would enable workers to advance up the skill and pay ladders.

The thrust of the foregoing has been to underscore that "the others," in particular physicians, hospitals, and hospital workers, benefited considerably, if indirectly, from the increased funding for improving and expanding health care for the elderly and the poor. In the section that follows we will probe further and suggest how the interests of "the others" came into conflict with improving the health care of the poor.

In the case of physicians, despite the considerable growth in the numbers practicing in the five boroughs, the low-income neighborhoods of the city were unable to make any significant progress in recruiting younger physicians. The reason is simply that the new reimbursement flows created a sufficient number of attractive career opportunities for U.S. medical school graduates in private practice and/or as members of AHCs and voluntary hospital staffs that physicians had no need to locate in areas where the poor lacked access. A related factor is that the abysmally low reimbursement rates under Medicaid were a serious deterrence to U.S. medical school graduates seeking to practice in New York City from locating in low-income neighborhoods.

_ The post-Medicare and Medicaid transformation of both the voluntary and public hospitals had other unanticipated consequences. Selected numbers of the poor had gained admission to the voluntary hospital system prior to the Medicare/Medicaid era because of their importance for teaching purposes. But with the passage of the new federal legislation the distinction between the poor and the nonpoor in terms of teaching material was eliminated with the result that the poor lost much of their earlier attractiveness to the teaching hospitals.

The greatly improved revenue position of most voluntary hospitals—particularly the major teaching hospitals—provided them with the opportunity to pursue their primary missions which did not include serious efforts to initiate new and improved ways of delivering health care services to the poor. Throughout the 1980s, the state commissioner of health, Dr. David Axelrod, pressured the medical leadership to establish community health centers in low-income neighborhoods for the purpose of enhancing the effectiveness of the medical care received by the poor. However, the medical leadership had other priorities for the expenditure of their enlarged revenue flows.

Although the HHC system ultimately decided to shift its focus from inpatient tertiary care to primary care for its essentially low-income patient constituency, the decline of the New York City economy and its tax levy revenues halted the implementation of the community health center effort (Communicare I) that it had initiated.

By way of summary: The elderly gained a great deal in improved access to quality mainstream care as a result of the passage of Medicare. In addition, those of the elderly who were on the margin of poverty or who required long-term care either in nursing homes or at home gained access via Medicaid to a much broadened range of essential health care services.

The blind and the disabled who had been largely neglected in the pre-Medicare/Medicaid era benefitted greatly when the federal government assumed responsibility via supplementary security income payments to cover their subsistence needs and provided them with wide ranging health care benefits—ambulatory, acute care hospitalization, nursing home care, and home care.

By far the largest group of Medicaid eligible persons in New York City, about six of ten, are the children and adults on AFDC and home relief who remain heavily dependent on the emergency rooms and clinics of the HHC for much of their ambulatory care, with other Medicaid eligibles using essential community providers or the voluntary hospital system's clinics and ERs. When it comes to inpatient care, the predominant number of the Medicaid eligible are treated in the voluntary system.

That leaves the most vulnerable of all the poor and the near poor, the uninsured—those who do not have private insurance and who cannot meet the eligibility requirements for Medicaid. While some of the uninsured obtain needed medical care from the voluntary hospital sector, for the most part they are heavily dependent on the HHC system for both ambulatory and inpatient services.

A balanced judgment about the city's poor is that many profited a great deal from the passage of Medicare and Medicaid, particularly the elderly, the blind, and the disabled; and that all of the poor had access to a higher level of care in 1995 than they had in 1965. However, it would be difficult to conclude there was a significant narrowing of the gap between the services available to the Medicaid population and the privately insured.

A case could be made that the greatest contribution to the city's poor from the post-1965 health care reforms were the substantial gains in hospital and related employment which expanded the job and income opportunities for many of the inner city residents, particularly poor minority women and many recent immigrants. Additional jobs and income probably contributed as much or more to the health of many of the poor than the expansion of health care services.

6

Innovative Programs

As previous chapters have indicated, the efforts to provide health care for the urban poor have undergone significant elaboration over the past thirty years. In this chapter we will examine some of the more significant programs that are now underway in New York City and assess their potential for improving health delivery for the poor. While few programs are designed explicitly to provide care for the uninsured, the programs discussed below all consider the needs of this group to be an integral part of their mission. In most cases, however, the care of the uninsured continues to be financed through subsidy and cross-subsidy from the care of other, better reimbursed patients. The impending decreases in health care funding that have been proposed in Congress as part of the federal budget for FY 1997 are likely to reduce the revenue base on which these subsidies depend. It is possible therefore that some time in the future many of the current experiments and demonstrations will be unable to continue to care for the uninsured. In the next chapter we will examine specifically the impact of Medicaid managed care.

Montefiore Medical Center and the Bronx Health Plan

The hospital most renowned for care of the poor in New York City is probably Montefiore Medical Center. Montefiore, more than any other hospital in New York, took advantage of federal programs from their onset in the 1960s. It was the first major medical center to operate an Office of Economic Opportunity Neighborhood Health Center, the Martin Luther King, Jr. (MLK) Center, which soon became the major noninstitutional provider of ambulatory care for poor and uninsured patients in the Bronx. Montefiore's leadership was critical for the establishment of new centers under other federal programs as well, including the Comprehensive Health Care Center (CHCC) and the Comprehensive Family Care Center (CFCC) run by the Albert Einstein College of Medicine (AECOM). The CFCC participated in Einstein's pathbreaking graduate medical education program in family medicine.

Montefiore was also a pioneer in the use of team approaches to family medical care when it launched the Valentine Lane Family Practice in south Yonkers, a demonstration initially supported by the Robert Wood Johnson Foundation. While not as successful as some of the hospital's larger ventures, many of the leaders of that program have gone on to distinguished careers in primary care medicine.

Perhaps the most significant contribution by Montefiore was its commitment to family and social medicine and the growth of residency programs in these areas. For most of the 1970s, the main training site for family medicine residents was St. Barnabas Hospital. When that institution decided to terminate all of its GME programs, Montefiore shifted them to its ambulatory care centers which became training grounds for the housestaff to an extent that no other medical school or hospital in New York has matched. The graduates of these programs became, in turn, the physicians who staffed the new ambulatory care centers that were being opened. This too was a significant development and differs from the experience of many other health centers operating under the auspices of a major teaching hospital or medical school. In most cases, graduates of the housestaff rarely stay on to become the full-time staff of the ambulatory centers, but at Montefiore this became the norm. At present Montefiore operates seven health centers including the CHCC, CFCC, MLK, and four small (5,000 sq. ft.) five-physician clinics. In all, the seven clinics had 232,000 visits in 1994. Sixty percent of the patients are on Medicaid, 6 percent on Medicare, and 34 percent are self-pay or uninsured. Current plans are to add another clinic by mid-1995 and four more by mid-1996.

Currently, the Montefiore clinics are training sixty-six primary care residents along with 176 third-year medical students serving six-week clerkships. There are also six nurse practitioner students doing fieldwork at the clinics. In order to ensure that GME monies go to Montefiore, the medical center owns the operating certificates of the ambulatory care centers. This represents the largest training effort in primary care in New York.

Montefiore, the private teaching hospital of AECOM, has benefited from the location of public hospitals proximate to its two campuses—

North Central Bronx Hospital is physically connected to the Moses (main) division of Montefiore, while Jacobi Hospital (Bronx Municipal Hospital) is across the street from the Weiler (Einstein) division. Both public hospitals are similarly major teaching facilities of Einstein. Uninsured and Medicaid patients can be transferred easily to the public institutions while the privately insured patients are treated in the private facilities. However, the same medical staff are responsible for treating all the patients in all the hospitals, a factor which has been associated with better outcomes for the poor patients. Montefiore has also benefited from a large volume of Medicare beneficiaries in its service area which has enabled the hospital to subsidize the care of the poor.

With a change in institutional leadership in the late 1970s, the hospital began to cut back its support of ambulatory care practice in the clinics. This decision has been reversed by the current administration and the program has, in fact, accelerated. In part the motive for this renewed interest in the promotion of primary care is the desire of the medical center to continue to play a prominent role in the health care delivery system of New York, but it is also a response to the new economics of medical care that makes primary care financially attractive. Moreover, the expansion of the hospital's primary care network widens the referral pool for filling the expensive inpatient beds of the medical center.

In a separate departure, the hospital began to plan a managed care program for Medicaid recipients as early as 1980. With support from the Commonwealth Fund, planning and development for a network of clinics that could provide a managed care package for Medicaid recipients was begun. It was not until 1985 that the necessary state approvals and waivers were granted and the program was operationalized. The plan, known as the Bronx Health Plan (BHP), now consists of the seven Montefiore clinics, the Morris Heights Health Center, and Soundview Health Center. The Montefiore clinics are responsible for 43 percent of the members. BHP is a not-for-profit entity licensed as a Primary Health Services Provider (PHSP) by New York State which permits it to provide services for Medicaid recipients only. It has become the largest provider of Medicaid managed care in the Bronx and has recently expanded to parts of Manhattan.

In essence, BHP is an administrative and marketing organization that contracts with clinic-based providers of primary care for services to Medicaid patients enrolled in managed care. The BHP receives capitation payments from Medicaid and makes arrangements with its constituent centers to provide care. The capitation rates that are paid to PHSPs average 89 percent of the average annual per capita cost (AAPCC) of the Medicaid program and while BHP gets a somewhat lower average, its efficiency allows it to generate a surplus that it feeds back into the centers.

The surplus from BHP makes up the operating deficit of the Montefiore centers which, given their high load of uninsured patients, are budgeted to lose money. Thus their participation in the plan allows the hospital to provide care for the uninsured without incurring financial risk. It should be noted that this use of the surplus also means that center growth must be supported from alternative funds. The long-standing system of cross-subsidization continues to operate in the U.S. hospital sector, although now ambulatory care operations are increasingly helping to subsidize inpatient care. While it is likely that the state will reduce the capitation payment for Medicaid managed care and thus reduce the ability of BHP to generate a surplus that helps to cover the uninsured, it is also likely that the expansion of BHP will attenuate this process somewhat. In the three and a half year period between May 1992 and October 1995, its enrollment has risen impressively, from 11,500 to 35,500.

This triad—training medical students and residents to work in urban primary care, providing hospital and medical care to a large number of uninsured, and operating a Medicaid HMO—makes the Montefiore system unique among New York City major medical centers and AHCs. In our judgment, Montefiore represents one of the best examples of the comprehensive integration of medical education with ambulatory and primary care delivery in the United States; the students who go through the program have been among the leaders of primary care medicine in the nation, particularly in terms of the care of the poor and uninsured. While other centers are beginning to emulate some of the same approaches, Montefiore has a long track record in this regard and remains a model to be followed.

Columbia-Presbyterian Medical Center and the Ambulatory Care Network Corporation (ACNC)

One of the most dramatic demographic changes in New York City took place in the areas of Washington Heights and Inwood, at the northernmost tip of Manhattan. What had been an enclave of the well-insured middle class, became the home of growing numbers of immigrants, primarily Dominicans, who were not insured.

The Latino community that accounts for almost two-thirds of the population is poor, with the lowest per capita income of any ethnic group in New York and correspondingly low employment rates. Moreover, language is a major barrier and a majority of the households do not have telephones. A recent survey indicated that fewer than 50 percent of the recently arrived residents of the area have health insurance, and since many are undocumented, access to Medicaid is low.

The birthrate in the area is 50 percent higher than for New York City as a whole and as a result, the pediatric population is also much higher than the rest of the city. Given the dismal socioeconomic indices of the population, its health status is surprisingly good. Nevertheless, it is a population with little access to appropriate medical care.

Presbyterian Hospital, the principal teaching hospital of the College of Physicians and Surgeons of Columbia University, is at present the sole provider of institutional care for the residents of the Washington Heights/Inwood area. Since 1967, eight acute care facilities with almost 1500 beds that served the area have closed and along with the bed closures there has been a decrease in the numbers of private practitioners willing to serve patients who are on Medicaid or uninsured. As a result, the Vanderbilt Clinic of Presbyterian Hospital receives over 500,000 ER and OPD visits a year and, given this volume of patients, it is not a tenable site for the provision of high quality, continuous, primary care.

Presbyterian is a major tertiary medical center with 971 beds occupying a new physical plant near the southern rim of Washington Heights/Inwood. The Allen Pavilion of Presbyterian Hospital is a stand-alone community hospital with 261 beds located about two miles from its parent facility. It was designed to handle the general acute care needs of the area and has a small outpatient department and emergency room that can accommodate only 20,000 visits per year.

The Ambulatory Care Network Corporation (ACNC) was established in 1985 to help ease the burden on Vanderbilt Clinic and the Presbyterian emergency room. It evolved from a series of community discussions about the future of health care in upper Manhattan following the demise of several nearby acute care facilities which left Presbyterian Hospital as the only institutional provider of care for a primary service area of almost 400,000 residents. The lack of private primary care physicians in the area was also a significant factor in the creation of the network. It is technically a demonstration project that operates with a three-year waiver from New York State (the waiver has been renewed three times). The ACNC is reimbursed through an experimental program called Products of Ambulatory Care (PACs) which is an analogue of inpatient DRGs applied to ambulatory care. The average per visit reimbursement to the ACNC is $105 which is about $30 higher than the reimbursement for an outpatient visit to the hospital. The ACNC clinics also operate at about half the actual cost of an outpatient visit. The corporation is designed to have six clinics (the last two are expected to open in 1996) located throughout the community that will provide primary care services to the population. In 1994 the four clinics in operation provided about 65,000 visits per year. The most recent clinic to open is an urgent care center located two city blocks from the main emergency room of Presbyterian Hospital. Transportation is provided for nonemergency patients to the center and once in the center the patients are registered in one of the primary care clinics. Through this mechanism the hospital hopes to lighten the load on its emergency room, to decrease its costs, and to promote the use of the primary care centers.

A major innovation being demonstrated in one of the ACNC clinics is the use of nurse practitioners to provide pediatric primary care. The demonstration is funded by the New York State Department of Health and entails the granting of full hospital admitting privileges for the nurse practitioners (NPs) who are permitted to follow the patients during their hospital stay and on their return, after discharge, to the primary care center. The program will be evaluated separately to determine whether NPs can provide high quality primary care at a lower cost or the same cost as physicians in a clinic setting. Also to be evaluated will be the productivity of the nurse practitioners in comparison with housestaff and salaried physicians. The demonstration should have much to contribute to the national debate on the role of nurses in primary care. Physicians are available for backup and referral should a case be deemed too complex by the NPs.

The ACNC clinics accept all patients regardless of ability to pay. It is less expensive for indigent patients to be treated on a comprehensive primary care basis than as emergency room patients and potential admissions to the Presbyterian Hospital. This is a major feature of the program, particularly in light of its setting in a community where lack of insurance is the norm. Social work staff at the clinics attempt to enroll patients who are eligible for the Medicaid program or to ascertain whether they have health care coverage of which they may not be aware, such as union-sponsored health insurance.

The aim of the ACNC is to provide community-based primary care using a staff of physicians and nurse practitioners. The physicians have admitting privileges at Presbyterian Hospital and Allen Pavilion and can follow their patients should they require hospital admission. Patients are assigned to a primary care provider and are given appointments with that provider. Although it is possible to have walk-in or emergency visits, such visits are discouraged in favor of telephone contact with the staff which is available around the clock. If an ACNC patient shows up at Vanderbilt Clinic or the ER at Presbyterian, the ACNC will be alerted and can either provide direct assistance to the patient or remind the patient of clinic procedures.

With the growth of Medicaid managed care and the high proportion of residents in northern Manhattan on Medicaid, it is reasonable to expect the ACNC to explore the provision of Medicaid managed care to its enrollees. The ACNC is currently affiliated with several commercial and not-for-profit HMOs in which the centers serve as the primary care providers for the HMOs. In addition, the ACNC has applied to New York State to become a Primary Health Services Provider (PHSP), the state designation for a Medicaid HMO. Although no final decision has yet been made on whether to become an HMO, the application, if approved, will enable the corporation to make that move should it be deemed advantageous. The ACNC provides care to the uninsured after making efforts to enroll members in Medicaid. As with the Bronx Health Plan, the surpluses that are generated from current Medicaid capitation rates help to subsidize the care of the uninsured. Moreover, the fact that treatment is less expensive at the ACNC and reimbursement is higher than it would be in a standard outpatient department also helps to lower the costs of treating the uninsured.

The ACNC is also working with community physicians to upgrade their practices and their medical skills. Community physicians who meet the qualifications of the medical staff are being given hospital admitting privileges and even medical school faculty appointments. The medical school has been awarded grants which allow it to train community physicians and to enhance their practice opportunities at both the hospital and the ACNC. Currently the ACNC is working with 200 physicians in the primary service area.

The longer-range goals for the ACNC are to attract private patients to the centers in addition to the current clientele of Medicaid enrollees and uninsured patients. The corporation also hopes to operate more in the model of a multispecialty group practice and to have community practitioners operate out of ACNC clinics. Of course, every clinic that caters to a primarily poor population hopes to expand its clientele to include the insured as well; if history is any judge, however, few of these efforts succeed. The ACNC stands out as a model for decreasing the dependence of a community on a large institutional facility and for educating a population accustomed to seek instant care at an emergency room, to use an appointment-based system. At present it is far less integrated with medical education than the Montefiore system, but it is planning to change. The medical school will be starting a family practice residency program based in Allen Pavilion that will utilize the ACNC centers as practice sites.

There are two major differences between the Montefiore model and the ACNC. The first is that the Montefiore model consists only of nonhospital based ambulatory care clinics while the ACNC includes the Vanderbilt Clinic as its major constituent. The off-hospital sites are attempts to reduce the utilization of the Vanderbilt OPD. Moreover, the ACNC holds the operating certificate for Vanderbilt Clinic: it is licensed by New York State as an Article 28 Diagnostic and Treatment Facility (DTF) and accordingly, Presbyterian Hospital has no outpatient department listed on its certificate of operation. The second difference is that Montefiore Medical Center owns the clinics that it operates in order to ensure that GME monies will go to the hospital. The ACNC is a separate corporation although Presbyterian Hospital still collects the GME money.

Lutheran Hospital

Lutheran Hospital has gained enviable distinction in the New York City health care sector as a result of its unusual origins and continued community activities. Once a failing institution in southwest Brooklyn, the hospital board was given a former bowling ball factory by the city of New York and financial support from the state of New York so that the interior of the facility could be gutted and redesigned as a modern hospital. Located in a heavily industrial area of Brooklyn and surrounded by few other health facilities, the hospital began to use its assets to assist the community.

Lutheran became famous for two things. A federally funded community health center (Sunset Park CHC) became the ambulatory department of the hospital and the hospital began a policy of upgrading its community. The hospital gave preference in hiring to community residents and encouraged its vendors to use community residents as workers also. Moreover, the hospital's development department began to apply for federal and state grants for different types of projects that would bring outside money into the hospital and the community. The hospital helped to build senior citizens housing and then provided medical care to the complex. The hospital hosted English-as-a-second-language (ESL) and general equivalency diploma (GED) programs to enhance the ability of neighborhood residents to get jobs. It was not long before the hospital was recognized as a leader in community relations by the American Hospital Association.

In 1984, the NYS DOH started a managed care demonstration program for the uninsured that covered services including mental health, alcoholism, and dentistry. The program paid $2 per member, per month. The purpose of the program was to see whether the state would save money by keeping people out acute care hospitals. As a result of the demonstration, the state began its Primary Health Service Provider (PHSP) program which was a precursor to the Medicaid Managed Care program.

In 1987, Lutheran responded to an RFP from the Robert Wood Johnson Foundation for Medicaid managed care demonstrations and was one of thirteen projects in the nation to be funded (along with the Bronx Health Plan). The three year grant allowed for the planning and administration of a managed care program for Medicaid recipients and included funding for an initial year of marketing in which the hospital sought to enroll 2,000 children in Child Health Plus. As part of this demonstration, the hospital received site-specific legislation and a HCFA waiver. The program that was established included dentistry, substance abuse, and mental health within the scope of primary care. It was targeted at the AFDC and SSI populations living adjacent to the hospital. However, there was little incentive for patients to enroll in the plan since they had to relinquish their Medicaid cards (and associated benefits) to join, and there was high disenrollment during the introductory phase. While it was clear that a mandatory managed care program would be useful, the city and state were not yet willing to commit to such a plan. As the cost of Medicaid continued to rise and word of experimentation with Medicaid managed care in other states reached New York, the decision was made to begin an experimental mandatory managed care program for Medicaid recipients.

On October 1, 1992 the new demonstration started in the southwest Brooklyn area broadly defined as Coney Island, Sheepshead Bay, Bensonhurst, and Sunset Park. The refusal of Coney Island Hospital to open a clinic meant that the program was focused around the Lutheran site. The waiver of section 1902 (a) (1) of the Social Security Act (Freedom of Choice in the Selection of Providers) allowing the demonstration to proceed was approved for a two year period to conclude on September 30, 1994. An evaluation of the program, performed by the New York State Department of Social Services, in order to have the waiver renewed for an additional two years (i.e. 1996), was quite promising. Although based on a small number of clients, the overall findings were as follows:

- Seventy-three percent of respondents were satisfied or very satisfied with their enrollment in the program and their access to care.
- The reasons given for disenrollment included having to use a physician who was not previously known to the patient; excessive travel time to the physician's office, and other logistic problems rather than outright dissatisfaction with the care.
- For a small sample of enrollees (100) and a matched control group from another area, the average monthly program cost came to $141.38 for the managed care recipients versus $147.64 for the fee-for-service recipients. It should be noted that there was no hospital expense for the managed care group during the study period.
- The overall compliance rate for well adult and child care, based on medical record audit, was 73 percent for the managed care group versus 46 percent for the fee-for-service comparison group. For sick child and adult care, the compliance rate was 87 percent for managed care versus 75 percent for fee-for-service.

In the southwest Brooklyn project, all AFDC Medicaid recipients must choose one of at least six managed care plans for their medical care unless they have either a well-established relationship with a particular provider or a chronic or mental health problem. At present the list consists of the following plans (PCPs): Aetna, Empire BC/BS HealthNet, Cigna, HIP, Lutheran Hospital Health Care Plus, and Oxford Health

Plan. While the project covers a large section of Brooklyn, Lutheran Hospital is the main institutional site of care. There are at least eight managed care plans competing for patients in the zip codes surrounding Lutheran including an HMO that Lutheran itself organized. In addition, Lutheran has become the site for a family medicine residency program which uses the Sunset Park Center as its clinical and training base.

Lutheran agreed to be the major participant in this demonstration for several reasons. As noted above, the hospital is managed by a forward-looking, progressive administration that is inclined to experiment with projects that might improve care to the community. In addition, Lutheran was noted for its ambulatory care programs, hence anything that would enhance this reputation would be useful for the entire hospital. The experience that Lutheran would gain as a demonstration site in the operation of a managed care program would give it a substantial advantage over other hospitals that would have to learn the same lessons but without state and federal support. Moreover, the hospital believed that even if the managed care experiment reduced inpatient admissions, acute care beds could be converted to care for patients with AIDS and alcoholism to make up for shortfalls.

As of 1995, 13,000 people had enrolled in the Lutheran Medical Center/Health Care Plus program. It has applied for a license as a PHSP to move into other areas and has formed a partnership with Sisters of Charity of Staten Island to serve all of Brooklyn and Staten Island; this will be a full capitation model with risk assumed by Sisters of Charity. The hospital also operates Child Health Plus, a Child Health Insurance Program (CHIP) with a current enrollment of about 5,000. In addition, Lutheran has signed an agreement with SUNY-Downstate Medical School to become its major affiliate for primary care. Residents in family practice will rotate through the entire Lutheran network and all the centers will become full primary care practice centers.

Over and above the activities noted above, Lutheran runs a freestanding family practice unit, a satellite for senior citizens in an American Legion Post, clinics in surrounding areas, an independent school health program for 11,000 children that generates 35,000 visits per year, a program with Pentecostal Church ministers to upgrade skills and referral patterns, and a similar program with the Chinatown Health Clinic in Manhattan since 40 percent of the patients who utilize that clinic live in Sunset Park.

Health and Hospitals Corporation Demonstration Projects

By far the most important source of care for the poor in New York City has long been the public hospital system which since 1979 has operated under the authority of the New York City Health and Hospitals Corporation (HHC).

The HHC has moved slowly and gradually from a traditional system of acute inpatient care and specialty outpatient clinics designed for the convenience of attending physicians and medical schools conducting clinical training, to a series of hospital-based primary care centers and increasing numbers of off-site primary care centers. Although most of the HHC activity has been dictated by the demands of Medicaid managed care (since Medicaid is responsible for 70 percent of the system's revenues), the changes are also having a dramatic impact on the care of the non-Medicaid poor and uninsured.

With the exception of trauma cases, very few people who utilize the public hospital system in New York have private physicians. Entry into the system is generally through an emergency room visit at which point triage takes place. Patients not in need of emergency care are generally referred to a clinic for treatment either the same day or some time later. The clinics generally do not have appointment systems (or effective appointment systems) and tend to operate on a first come-first serve basis. After a wait that may take several hours, patients are either sent to a hospital pharmacy for medication, if indicated, or given a return appointment for the same or a different clinic. These encounters may last as long as four to six hours and may require movement between the clinic and ancillary service centers. Follow-up visits may be compromised by the inability to retrieve prior medical records, change in the provider of care (i.e., different medical staff or residents), or the need to utilize services not available at that particular time or location. This inefficiency, long noted, serves to increase costs greatly, decrease patient satisfaction, and engender ill will towards the public system. This is intensified by the sheer volume of patient visits on any given day in a system that provides nearly 6 million (1994) visits per year.

The acknowledgment that this has not been a particularly effective method of providing care has not meant that it has undergone substantial change. What has generally happened is that each time a new administration has attempted to address the problem, funding cuts or other crises have intervened to make reform of ambulatory care delivery a back burner issue. The process actually started to change in the early 1980s during a period of managerial stability, friendly relations with the mayor's office, and a primary care-minded president of the HHC. Some hospital clinics were converted into primary care centers, new Neighborhood Family Care Centers (large primary care clinics) were established and attempts were made to reform the patient scheduling and appointment process. By the late 1980s, many of these efforts were again relegated to back-burner status as a new administration and a new mayor sought to make different changes in the way the hospitals and clinics functioned.

The overwhelming impact of Medicaid managed care on HHC revenues and the realization that voluntary sector providers were beginning to court patients who had formerly been restricted to the HHC, gave impetus to a new movement for change. The first development was the decision to convert former Department of Health categorical clinics into primary care centers and to transfer their management to the HHC. This process which has taken several years to implement has thus far had mixed results. On the one hand, simply calling a clinic a primary care center does not make it one. Since most of the personnel who now work in the clinics were part of the older system, and since the imperatives of medical education did not change, the ability to provide continuity of care, centralized and computerized medical records, and accurate patient appointment scheduling did not automatically change. Over time a growing cadre of HHC workers has learned how to provide primary care, the investments in computerized medical records systems and computer scheduling software have been productive, and perhaps most important, changes in medical school affiliation contracts have led to a greater emphasis on primary care.

Several problems still remain. Many of the clinics, while suitable for primary care services, must send patients to a tertiary hospital for specialized diagnostic and therapeutic services. It is at this point that the model fails since the scheduling and team concepts and the ability to return patients to the originating center do not work very well. Moreover, it is confusing for patients to have to deal with totally different approaches to medical care delivery within the same organization.

It has been difficult for HHC to insist that patients remain attached to one delivery site. Patients can always go to whatever hospital and clinic they choose and know they will not be turned away. As a result substantial patient education for optimal utilization of the primary care services that are available is needed, but it has been difficult to operationalize.

In 1991, the Communicare plan was officially announced by Mayor David Dinkins. Communicare was essentially a formalization of the attempts to turn categorical clinics into primary care centers. As initially proposed, thirty clinics were to be converted over a relatively short period of time using monies from the city's capital budget. However, there were no plans for new staff training, the hiring of new providers, and other noncapacity-related issues. The management structure for the new centers was also left relatively loose. Communicare was superseded by a new effort designated Communicare II which sought to convert a total of sixty clinics to primary care centers. As this process got underway, the usual panoply of factors that affect a public hospital system came into play—a new administration with a different set of priorities, a substantial structural deficit in the city's budget which was to be addressed by large scale cuts in the city's payment to HHC, and the retirement or buy-out of a large number of senior staff members. The central office of the HHC was a featured target in budget cutting and although this was perceived as preferable to cutting frontline personnel in the hospitals and clinics, it has made it difficult to implement the new primary care initiatives.

The attempt to enroll patients in the HHC Medicaid HMO, Metropolitan Health Plus, has also been given precedence over the need to enhance the primary care infrastructure. With a shrinking sum of money to accomplish the various needs of the public hospital system, primary care infrastructure has become a luxury rather than an absolute priority. The continuing threat to the HHC budget both from federal and state cuts in Medicaid and, perhaps most of all, from Mayor Giuliani's desire to privatize HHC and take the city out of the business of health services delivery, has also contributed to the difficulty of recruiting a stable staff capable of implementing the changes required to establish a first-class primary care system.

The Capital Needs for Primary Care Delivery

New York City hospitals have long been dependent on the FHA hospital bond insurance program in order to access the capital markets. Even hospitals in the most affluent areas of the city have below average financial indicators and ratios and therefore find it difficult to sell their bonds without some form of insurance. As was noted in a previous chapter, the substandard operating statistics are largely related to the unique hospital financing system used in New York State and must therefore be interpreted with caution. Low operating margins do not necessarily indicate that a hospital is in financial trouble so much as that its potential to increase revenues is limited by the absence of cost shifting. Margins can also be lower than those of hospitals in other states since the revenues that hospitals receive include payment for uncompensated care and capital pass-throughs. The subtleties of New York City hospital operating statistics aside, investment bankers have been able to sell New York City hospital debt only by guaranteeing the payment of principle and interest through the use of bond insurance that has been available solely through the federal government's program. It is worth noting that 86 percent of the FHA portfolio is in New York City hospital bonds.

There are some hospitals whose bonds even the FHA will not insure; these tend to be the voluntary hospitals that are located in areas where the poorest New Yorkers live. The bulk of the patient revenues in these hospitals is generated by the uninsured and Medicaid recipients and most of them live with negative fund balances and negative financial indicators. In many cases these are hospitals that in an earlier time relied on community philanthropy that no longer exists as the population demographics have changed and the philanthropic agencies have shifted their support to other institutions. Yet these are clearly needed hospitals and they tend to be the sole community providers of care in areas with few private physicians and a lack of other medical resources.

New York State adopted a unique approach to dealing with this problem by creating the fiscally distressed hospitals capital fund. In essence, the NYPHRM system allows hospitals to be designated "fiscally distressed" and as such they are fully reimbursed for their uncompensated care revenues. Yet even under these circumstances the capital markets refused to accept bonds issued for these institutions (or more accurately, there were no buyers for such bonds). Without access to the capital markets, the hospitals were unable to improve their efficiency, upgrade their standards to meet changing health and safety codes, or buy new equipment. The hospitals would have been forced to close once their accreditation was withdrawn as a result of these deficiencies.

New York's solution was to create a mechanism that offered these hospitals access to a special capital pool backed by the moral authority of New York State. A revolving fund was created by the New York State

Medical Care Facilities Financing Authority (MCFFA) which permitted fiscally distressed institutions to apply for monies for capital renovation and modernization. Special assurances were provided to guarantee that the hospitals could pay back the bonds, but in the case of default, they would be backed up by New York State. The technical name for this type of financing is "service obligations," but it would also be accurate to refer to them as "moral obligation" bonds, since they are not backed by any collateral other than the reputation of the state.

This method has proven effective as a means of ensuring that hospitals serving the poorest New Yorkers can remain in good condition and meet upgraded safety standards. However, there has been no mechanism that would allow smaller facilities to tap the capital markets. Despite the need to increase primary care capacity in New York City, no ready source of funding to do so is available. These problems were particularly acute for clinics that sought to expand their current capacity or to make structural changes in order to provide primary care services more efficiently. Further, it was feared that if Medicaid patients selected facilities based on amenities and modernization, for-profit centers and managed care companies with access to the equity market would place nonprofit and public facilities at a competitive disadvantage. As a result, the Primary Care Development Corporation (PCDC), an analogue to the fiscally distressed hospitals capital fund, was established.

PCDC was given initial support from philanthropies and city monies which enabled it to create a revolving capital fund with the cooperation of the MCFFA. RFPs were issued to identify ambulatory care providers in New York City who would be interested in applying for new capital funds to renovate existing space or expand their physical capacity to provide new primary care services. The first PCDC selection cycle (1994) designated nineteen projects to receive a total $91 million. The majority (thirteen) were for new facilities, the rest (six) for expansion or relocation. Overall they will add almost 700,000 new visits to an existing total of about 350,000 (table 6.1).

With this mechanism in place, the ability of smaller voluntary clinics, community health centers, and other health care providers to improve their physical capacity to provide primary care is enhanced. In addition to capacity building, PCDC is also interested in ensuring that its recipients (and others) acquire management education, financial planning and budgeting skills, greater knowledge about primary care and

TABLE 6.1
Primary Care Development Corporation (PCDC) Projects—1994 Selection Cycle

Sponsor	Location	Estimated New Visits	Project Type*
Institute for Urban Family Health	Bronx	17,500	N
Urban Health Plan, Inc.	Bronx	45,000	Exp
Morris Heights Health Center	Bronx	43,000	N
Bronx-Lebanon Hospital	Bronx	18,000	N
Promesa D+TC	Bronx	22,417	Exp
Narco Freedom	Bronx	36,000	N
North Bronx Health Center	Bronx	58,655	N
Bedford-Stuyvesant Family Health Center	Brooklyn	75,000	Exp
Caribbean Women's Health Association	Brooklyn	30,000	N
Brooklyn Hospital Center	Brooklyn	52,000	N
Lutheran Medical Center	Brooklyn	20,000	Exp
Settlement Health and Medical Service, Inc.	Manhattan	30,000	Exp
Community Family Planning	Manhattan	10,600	N
Community Health Project, Inc	Manhattan	30,912	Exp
Presbyterian ACNC	Manhattan	101,625	N
Boriken Neighborhood Health Center	Manhattan	17,000	N
Mary Immaculate Hospital	Queens	37,000	N
St. John's Episcopal Hospital	Queens	20,000	N
St. Vincent's, Staten Island	Staten Island	16,800	N

* N=new; Exp=expansion

Source: Primary Care Development Corporation, November 1994

how it should work, and skills and techniques in professional development. It sees itself not only as a funder but also as a resource center for primary care.

Because PCDC has only a limited amount of money with which to finance new projects, its ability to increase capacity beyond a certain point is severely constrained. There is no question that the need for primary care centers in New York goes well beyond what PCDC could fund even over a multiyear period.

It has been estimated that the average cost of establishing a small primary care center is $1 million. While this is not a major challenge for a large hospital, it does represent a significant sum for a community clinic. Moreover, in a period when health care reimbursement is declining, the outlay of even relatively small amounts of money for new ventures may easily be second-guessed. Thus, a number of hospitals are in the process of contracting with existing for-profit managed care firms to develop new clinic capacity that would be financed by the managed care firms, whose patients, in return, would have first access to the facilities.

These ventures are likely to produce substantial growth in the city's nonhospital based primary care capacity. However, this represents only one factor in the provision of primary care—structural capacity. The complementary factor—ensuring that there is an adequate supply of primary care physicians who will provide care—is a far more complicated issue because of the long period of time required to train new primary care practitioners.

All of the facilities that receive support through PCDC provide some service to Medicaid recipients. Here again, developing the human resources component of primary care is problematic because managed care companies that have no obligation to treat the uninsured are in the best position to recruit qualified physicians and other personnel.

While several of the medical schools in New York City have begun to establish departments of family medicine or primary care and to develop corresponding residency programs, the small numbers of students involved at present and the long training period mean that these initiatives will not have a serious impact on the delivery of primary care in New York for many years to come.

Of the roughly 25,000 physicians who are licensed to practice and designate New York City as their practice location, only about 7,500 claim to practice primary care. As of late 1994, approximately 2,000 of these physicians participated in for-profit managed care organizations along with approximately 500 subspecialists who also served as primary care providers in these organizations. The remaining 5,500 primary care doctors may or may not join managed care plans, and may or may not elect to serve Medicaid patients in these plans. Totally lacking at present are primary care physicians in private practice who are willing to care for the poor and the uninsured.

Medical recruiters report that as the demand for primary care physicians has increased, the salaries offered to obtain these physicians has increased as well. Moreover, with a nationwide demand for primary care doctors, the ability of New York City to compete for these scarce resources is limited. Although institutional providers may be able to offer packages of incentives, salary, and amenities that would attract a primary care physician to New York, it is unlikely that community health centers and similar organizations are in a comparable position. As the cost of employing a primary care doctor increases, the employing institution is likely to seek a greater financial return from the physician. This would imply that the physician's practice time should be more gainfully spent, that is, with patients for whom they will be reimbursed.

Perhaps the best likelihood for increasing the numbers of physicians in New York City who could provide effective primary care will come from the retraining of specialists and subspecialists. Specialists are finding their services in less demand as managed care enrollment increases across the city. Many would like to continue practicing medicine but are no longer familiar with the elements of primary care needed to function as gatekeepers in a managed care system.

The New York State Department of Health has started a demonstration project aimed at retraining specialists to become certified as primary care doctors. How to ensure that these physicians treat not only patients for whom they are reimbursed but also the uninsured remains problematic.

The wide variety of demonstrations, experiments, and new ventures that are currently being implemented in New York City represent the late start that the city has gotten in meeting the need to provide noninstitutional services to the poor. The attempts to change have been complicated by the pressing needs on the institutional side and the difficulties of getting entrenched bureaucracies to move expeditiously. In this sense, New York has made phenomenal progress; however, much remains to be accomplished. As the ranks of the uninsured grow and as fiscal stringency begins to erode the ability of institutional providers to care for the uninsured and the non-Medicaid poor, the problems inherent in dealing with this population will become more apparent.

The U.S. Supreme Court issued a unanimous opinion in May 1995 which upheld the right of the state to set hospital rates without violating the ERISA law. This victory for rate setting and for the ability to tax the payers for care to provide reimbursement for the uninsured represents a major victory for the state, but one that is threatened by other factors.

Unless renewed, NYPHRM, the rate setting system that sets hospital inpatient rates and creates the bad debt and charity care pool which allows hospitals to care for the uninsured, will expire in June, 1996. Whether this will happen is uncertain. However the state now has a conservative governor who believes in the free market rather than regulation, a substantial part of the revenues in New York State are now outside this regulated system (e.g., Medicare and managed care which do not contribute to the pools represent about 45 percent of current inpatient revenues), and the managed care organizations that have become major powers in health policy in the past few years have no interest in the system. If there is no hospital rate regulation, there will be a severe challenge to state and city government to create a new mechanism that will allow for the continuing care of the poor.

In addition to this major problem at the state level, there is the expectation of substantial cuts in Medicare and Medicaid funding at the federal level which will crimp the ability of hospitals to subsidize the care of the poor. Although we cannot predict the outcome of future federal action, as of mid-1995 it was estimated that New York City could lose on the order of $33 billion over a seven year period in Medicaid and Medicare funding from the federal government.

Finally, and perhaps most directly relevant, is the future of the Health and Hospitals Corporation in New York. The current mayor, Rudolph Giuliani, has declared that the city has no business providing hospital services. The recent (August, 1995) *Report of the Advisory Panel on the Future of the Health and Hospitals Corporation*, issued by a task force that he established, called for the total elimination of the public hospital system in New York. The report states that the care of the uninsured should be the responsibility of the state or the federal government rather than the city and that the city can no longer afford this cost. Although the report has engendered much controversy and it is not clear what the ultimate outcome will be or what the politics of attempting to close the HHC might entail, the movement does not bode well for the poor and their health care needs.

The absence of universal health insurance in the United States, which also seems likely to continue for at least the rest of the decade, is the major risk factor in the way of delivering effective health care services to the poor. New York City has done much over the years to accommodate to this situation, but it may be that in a constricted, free market health care system it will no longer be possible to do so.

7

Medicaid Managed Care

The first systematic attempt to enroll Medicaid recipients in a managed care plan in New York City came in the early 1980s as part of an effort to bail out Metropolitan Hospital, a municipal facility that had been slated for closing in a budget-cutting strategy of Mayor Ed Koch. Community opposition to the closing led to the search for alternative approaches, among them the development of a managed care plan for both Medicaid-eligible and uninsured residents of the area surrounding the hospital. This effort was assisted by funding from both the federal and state governments that allowed the hospital to stay open. The state legislature, however, while granting money for a small demonstration at the hospital, refused to enact a program that would restrict Medicaid recipients in the area to the exclusive use of that one facility. The loss of "freedom of choice" was seen as a serious defect, and the legislature acceded only to a small demonstration project. The Metropolitan Health Plan, as it was called, never had more than 5,000 members and has since been folded into the MetroPlus plan run by the Health and Hospitals Corporation.

The Health Insurance Plan (HIP), a large group model HMO that had been in operation in New York since the mid-1940s, also began an experiment in which Medicaid recipients could enroll in the HMO rather than continue with fee-for-service Medicaid. The HIP program was successful and attracted over 40,000 Medicaid recipients with little fanfare.

Between 1980 and 1991, there were several other small Medicaid managed care demonstrations around New York State, sponsored by hospitals, medical societies, and academic health centers, mostly with the support of private philanthropies.

It has long been a commonplace that states serve as laboratories of democracy and as worksites for the development and testing of new approaches to traditional ideas. This certainly seems to be the case in New York State.

In 1991, confronted by the most expensive Medicaid program in the country, the New York State legislature passed the Medicaid Managed Care Act (Chapter 165 of the Laws of 1991) which mandated the voluntary enrollment of 50 percent of the state Medicaid population in managed care plans by 1997. This move was inspired by the actions of other states that had introduced Medicaid managed care, the particular ways that Medicaid recipients obtain health care in New York, and the need to improve quality and lower the cost of care. For New York City, the law would have meant the enrollment of almost 800,000 people in managed care within five years.

At the time, only a small minority of the Medicaid recipients in the state were members of managed care plans, the vast majority of these in the Health Insurance Plan (HIP) in New York City. If other states could benefit by moving their Medicaid populations into managed care, the argument went, this strategy could also apply to New York.

An additional factor that appealed to the legislature was the ability of managed care, at least in theory, to alter the way that people receive care. The Medicaid recipients of New York, particularly New York City, have sought care largely from hospital outpatient departments and emergency rooms, arguably the most expensive modalities of health care delivery. The New York City Health Systems Agency pioneered in the identification of "ambulatory care sensitive conditions" (ACSC), conditions that would not require hospitalization if the patient obtained timely primary care services. In a review of hospital records, Medicaid beneficiaries in New York City were found to have a disproportionate frequency of ACSC admissions. By stressing primary care, the legislature believed, managed care might be able to reorient the way that care was provided in New York, thereby reducing its cost and improving its quality.

The hallmark of the episodic treatment of Medicaid enrollees in hospital-based outpatient settings was noncontinuous, noncomprehensive, and noncost-effective care. Managed care offered the possibility not only of moving the locus of care but also of changing the way care was delivered by providing designated primary care physicians, accessible medical records, scheduled appointments, and an effective health team including nurse practitioners and a range of other paraprofessional personnel. This mechanism to improve the quality of care was also appealing to the members of the legislature tired of spending large sums of money with little return in terms of improved services and results.

Of course, the legislature would have been loath to consider any of this if not for the fact that managed care promised to lower the costs of the Medicaid program in addition to all of the other benefits. The basic formula was that an HMO would be paid 95 percent of the average annual per capita cost (AAPCC) to Medicaid and therefore, other things being equal, the state would save 5 percent through the use of managed care. As the program continued, the payments could be ratcheted down and additional sums saved. Since the Medicaid caseload was expected to increase, the shift to managed care would enable the state to avoid expanding its budgetary commitment to Medicaid expenditures.

Realizing that it was proposing a major change in the way that care was delivered and that considerable lead time would be needed to develop the physical capacity and the personnel to provide the managed care services and to establish the regulatory infrastructure, the legislature proposed a five-year target period in which to enroll 50 percent of the Medicaid population in managed care programs across the state. The program has been deemed successful as measured by the consistent growth in enrollments and the low level of complaints from either providers or Medicaid recipients. Table 7.1 indicates its progress in terms of participating plans and enrollments in New York City.

TABLE 7.1
Medicaid Managed Care Enrollment in New York City, 5/92–10/31/95

Managed Care Plan	Enrollment		
	5/92	*10/31/94*	*10/31/95*
HIP/99	40,218	59,416	63,244
HIP/O2	0	17,389	18,693
HIP-BI/LINK	0	79	57
Elderplan	123	132	125
Bronx Health Plan (PHSP)	11,473	27,998	35,561
Manhattan PHSP	3,836	12,897	27,875
Lutheran Health Plus Prepaid Health Services	4,781	10,223	13,712
Metropolitan Health Plan	3,891	23,956	69,515

TABLE 7.1 (continued)
Medicaid Managed Care Enrollment in New York City, 5/92–10/31/95

Managed Care Plan		Enrollment	
	5/92	*10/31/94*	*10/31/95*
US Healthcare, Inc.	348	28,358	34,434
Aetna Health Plans of NY, Inc.	0	1,418	1,461
Empire BC/BS Healthnet	0	2,810	2,608
Oxford Health Plans, Inc.	0	30,531	47,796
Healthcare of NY, Inc. Cigna	0	2,532	3,018
Beth Abraham Comprehensive Care Management	87	240	321
Primecare	0	5,381	933
Managed Healthcare Systems	0	25,828	46,131
Staten Island PCP	0	260	704
Catholic Health Services Plan	0	11,334	25,396
Healthfirst PHSP, Inc.	0	935	43,917
The New York Health Plan, Inc.	0	0	17,687
St. Barnabas Community Health Plan	0	0	1,956
Metlife (HMO)	0	0	158
Universal Health Plan	0	0	1,428
Neighborhood Health Providers	0	0	1,556
Wellcare of New York, Inc.	0	0	5,884
Managed Health, Inc.	0	2,337	3,012
Total enrollment	*64,762*	*264,054*	*467,182*

The law also created a new category of provider, a Prepaid Health Services Provider (PHSP) designated specifically to enroll Medicaid recipients. At present, 26 PHSPs are operating in New York City.

In addition to the statewide voluntary program, New York City obtained a 1902 (a) (1) waiver (Freedom of Choice in the Selection of Provider) from HCFA to conduct a mandatory managed care demonstration for Medicaid recipients in a defined area in Brooklyn. The southwest Brooklyn project, as it is known, has been in operation since October 1992 and is described in detail in chapter 6 (Innovative Programs) as one of the major efforts of Lutheran Hospital which is its institutional base.

With the election of Governor George Pataki in 1994, and the need to cut Medicaid spending in the face of an impending $4 billion-plus budget shortfall, the new administration proposed a waiver from the federal government that would permit compulsory enrollment in managed care programs of the state's entire Medicaid population. Technically, the state requested an 1115 waiver from the Health Care Finance Administration (HCFA) in order to enroll 85 percent of all Medicaid recipients in managed care plans within a two-year period and to enroll people with HIV/AIDS and mental health problems in so-called special needs plans (SNPs) to be established. The waiver also calls for converting the 100 percent state-financed home relief category of Medicaid into a federal participating category eligible for matching funds and disproportionate share funding. The purpose of this was to lock in additional federal funding in anticipation of the shift to federal block grants for the Medicaid program. In addition to the 1115 waiver proposed by the state, New York City has proposed a 1915-b waiver which would convert the entire AFDC Medicaid population of New York City from a fee-for-service program to a mandatory managed care program. This waiver was subsequently denied by HCFA, although the state waiver is still pending.

These proposals represent a dramatic departure from the more gradual, phased-in approach to managed care that New York had been pursuing. Moreover, the problems inherent in this more precipitous approach would create a significant set of issues for both the state and the city which are worth examining since they apply to all the states that are relying on managed care to rescue their Medicaid programs.

The most important question revolves around capacity to deliver primary care—both physical capacity, that is, offices and clinics, and personnel, specifically providers of primary care. Since New York intends to enroll some 2 million Medicaid beneficiaries (over 1.6 million in New York City) in managed care expeditiously, the issue is of some urgency. The projections of enrollment throughout the state noted in the proposed waiver application are as follows:

TABLE 7.2
Projected Enrollment in Medicaid Managed Care in New York State

Month/Year	Total	Increment
Actual (2/95)	500,000	
May, 1996	1,200,000	700,000
November, 1996	1,700,000	500,000
May, 1997	2,400,000	700,000
November, 1997	2,900,000	500,000
May, 1998	3,200,000	300,000
Total New Enrollment		2,700,000

Note: Includes projected growth in Medicaid case load. Enrollment complete in May, 1998.

Inasmuch as each enrollee in the program will be provided with a primary care physician whom, it is expected, the patient should be able to see within a reasonable period of time, an extraordinary expansion of capacity will be required. Since submission of the waiver application to HCFA, the stae has decelerated its enrollment schedule as a result of irregularities and deficiencies in the recruiting practices of the managed care organizations. Nevertheless, the rapid recruitment of the needed supply of generalists remains a crucial issue, regardless of targeted enrollment dates.

As we noted earlier, New York City has increased its primary care visit capacity through various mechanisms over the past several years, but even this growth will not be adequate to meet the needs of the large numbers of Medicaid patients who will shift from fee-for-service to managed care. The first round of facility construction funded by the Primary Care Development Corporation (PCDC) will add 681,509 visits to the current primary care capacity of the city but it will be several years before this new capacity will actually come on-line since construction has not yet started. A list of the projects is found in chapter 6, table 6.1.

All of the PCDC projects are being undertaken by not-for-profit organizations and hospitals. For-profit managed care companies are also expanding their capacity to participate in the Medicaid managed care program by constructing new clinics and by contracting with existing clinics for use of their facilities. While not intended exclusively for the use of the Medicaid population, all the PCDC sites must accept Medicaid patients. It seems likely that the for-profit clinics now under construction are planned exclusively for the Medicaid population so there will be no mixing of the Medicaid clientele with commercially insured patients.

The population specified in the Medicaid waiver includes some of the most severely ill people in the city—the homeless, Home Relief enrollees, and SSI beneficiaries whom the state also proposes to enroll expeditiously in managed care plans. For various reasons, the AFDC segment of Medicaid (numerically the largest) is relatively easy to transfer: it is possible to calculate their average cost per member per month and it is a relatively healthy population, particularly when provided with primary care in the form of prenatal services and postnatal well baby care. In the case of the other groups, the situation is very different. It is not at all clear how the homeless will be assigned to particular providers and how appointments will be scheduled. The amount of care that it will be necessary to provide to this group is substantial and the prospects of preventive care are minimal. The Home Relief population consists in large part of substance abusers who may also require substantial amounts of care. It may turn out that providers will not pursue these groups too assiduously as they are likely to be far less profitable than the AFDC Medicaid recipients. The essential point is that it is difficult to calculate in advance an adequate primary care capacity (in terms of visits) for populations that have never been enrolled in managed care programs. This problem is especially pertinent for New York City where reliance on institutionally provided care has been high and where the conversion process is likely to be difficult.

Thus far we have addressed the problem of ensuring adequate physical capacity to provide primary care. Although it would be useful to have clinics and offices in which primary care can be effectively provided, the reality is that much of the primary care encounters will continue to take place in outpatient departments and emergency rooms. A intrinsic more profound problem, which has no easy solution, is ensuring the provider capacity to deliver primary care services to this population.

New York City physicians, as we have noted, have never participated to any significant degree in the Medicaid program largely because the reimbursement was so low. In addition, physicians who did participate found that they were subject to audit by the state and generally had to wait several months before receiving any payment for their services. The rates were initially set low, in part because physicians had shown no great enthusiasm for the program and in part because poor people had traditionally been cared for in hospital OPDs and ERs and these institutions were reluctant to have more of the Medicaid funds channeled to physicians. Having set the preconditions for failure to attract physicians to the program, the state was never in a position to change its spending mode so as to increase the amount physicians received. Over time, as the differential between market fees and Medicaid reimbursement widened, the participation of private physicians declined further. Moreover, hospitals became even more reliant on the outpatient reimbursement from Medicaid and exercised their influence to dissuade legislators from increasing the payments to physicians for treating Medicaid patients.

It has been estimated that no more than 15 to 20 percent of the doctors in New York City (approximately 4 to 5,000) actually billed the program at any point in time for services rendered and many of them indicated institutional addresses (i.e., clinics) rather than private offices. Now that the program is moving to a managed care mode of delivery which is dependent on the provision of services by physicians, it is far from certain that an adequate number of doctors willing to treat Medicaid patients is available. Every analysis of physician location and poverty in New York has found an inverse relationship between poverty level and physician presence. Since primary care depends on convenient access to a physician, to make the system work there will be a need for substantial physician relocation. While it may be possible to increase the numbers of offices and clinics in areas where the Medicaid population live, it may not be easy to find physicians who are willing to work in those clinics and provide the needed care.

A related issue is the need for a sufficient supply of primary care physicians. Primary care, conventionally defined, consists of internal medicine, family practice, pediatrics, and ob-gyn. Using this definition, only about 30 percent of the doctors in New York classify as primary care practitioners. The growth of managed care—Medicaid, Medicare, and private—heightens the need for primary care physicians substantially; how they will be recruited is problematic.

The academic debates over the provision of primary care services have raged, unresolved, for the past thirty-five years. This is a particularly acute problem in the case of New York City because of the need to adapt rapidly to the needs of a very large group of Medicaid recipients, not to mention the commercially insured population. In the past, many different strategies have been tried to lure physicians to practice in low income areas in the city and almost all have been unsuccessful. Although no one thus far has attempted the rewards approach, that is, making Medicaid a better paying proposition, it seems unlikely that the needed number of physicians can be secured within the framework laid out by the waiver application.

There are three basic reasons why this seems to be the case. First, there is an overall shortage of primary care doctors being produced both in New York and nationally; second, reimbursement has not been nearly adequate to sustain a physician in a poor community without substantial subsidization from insured patients; and third, even if there were an adequate number of well-paid primary care physicians, they might not be inclined to practice in poor communities. Let us consider these problems in turn.

New York City has six medical schools within its boundaries and a seventh not far to the north that maintains its major teaching hospitals within the city. With the exception of Albert Einstein College of Medicine, these schools have avoided sponsoring primary care residency programs and promoting primary care, preferring instead to concentrate on research and subspecialty medicine. The absence of a strong base of managed care in New York City and the presence of such large numbers of specialists have meant that there has been no particular need for primary care doctors. Insured patients have been able to consult the specialist(s) of their choice and have felt confident that they could always be referred to another specialist should their medical management warrant it. Moreover, there is no real shortage of physicians trained in the primary care specialties in New York, and it is not difficult to find a general internist or pediatrician if one lives in an affluent community. New York City accounts for 14 percent of all the physicians trained in the United States and exports most of them to less doctored areas, very likely because the more attractive practice locations are already saturated and new graduates seeking to establish a career can find better opportunities elsewhere.

Even if all the medical schools were to reorient their educational objectives and develop residency programs in the primary care disciplines, the long period of training would mean that the graduates would not be available to the market in less than five to ten years. It would be possible to train other primary care health providers such as nurse practitioners or physician assistants in a shorter period of time; however, their high cost and lingering consumer skepticism of their efficacy suggest that they cannot compensate completely for this deficiency. Although there may be adequate numbers of medical students trained as primary care physicians in the future, meeting the needs of massive managed care enrollments right now is an urgent challenge.

The second issue confronting provider capacity for Medicaid managed care derives from the proposition, held by many, that the problem is essentially maldistribution. There are ample numbers of doctors in affluent, well-insured areas of the city but a dearth in areas of poverty and Medicaid concentration. Paradoxically, New York City has over one physician for every 500 residents (far better than the national average) yet half of all New Yorkers live in federally designated Health Professions Shortage Areas (HPSAs) and Medically Underserved Areas (MUAs). The criterion for designation as an HPSA is a physician to population ratio of less than one doctor per 3,500 people. Studies in New York have found that in central Harlem there is less than one physician for every 10,000 people, in stark contrast to the upper east side of Manhattan where there is over one physician for every sixty people.

By itself, this maldistribution is not necessarily a problem. New York City is not exceptionally dispersed geographically, it has excellent mass transportation, and in general people living in one area of a borough do not have too much trouble reaching another. The fact that most physicians in New York do not treat Medicaid patients means that even with proximity to physician-rich areas, there is no assurance that a person who is poor or on Medicaid can find a doctor to provide care. This contributes to the great use of institutional facilities for primary care in New York.

From the inception of the Medicaid program, it was clear that there was a way for physicians to game the system to maximize their revenues. While the unit payments by Medicaid were low, a high volume of services could generate a substantial income. The Medicaid mills that were established shortly after the program came into existence exploited communities with high Medicaid concentrations, using a strategy of ping-ponging patients among their specialist members and encouraging frequent visits to generate large revenues. When New York State began to crack down on the mills, it became apparent that they were the only providers of care to the poor in some neighborhoods and without them, patients were forced to use hospitals for all their care resulting in even higher costs to the Medicaid program. An attempt was made to work with the mills, renamed shared health facilities, in order to improve the quality of care rendered by them, but these efforts faltered due to lack of interest on the part of their physician members in obtaining admitting privileges at hospitals, enrolling in continuing medical education courses, or providing enhanced services. When the state health and social services officials finally realized that these efforts were doomed to failure, they redirected their strategy for improved service delivery for the poor to the academic medical centers whom they encouraged to provide off-site care in underserved communities.

Most of the physicians who practice in the Medicaid mills are international medical graduates (IMGs). In many cases English is not their primary language and they have substantial difficulties communicating with patients (who often don't speak English as a primary language either, but neither do they speak the language the doctor does). The IMGs have not been able to create successful practices in the privately insured sector, and as a result have tended to work in poor communities where the patients have little choice of provider.

As for U.S.-trained physicians, given the average level of debt that they have incurred prior to starting a practice, it is not realistic to expect them to practice in areas where they will be unable to maintain the lifestyle they aspire to if the majority of their patients are on Medicaid or are uninsured. Attempts to homestead physicians in underserved areas of New York have foundered for this reason, even when doctors have been guaranteed an income, loan repayment, malpractice coverage, and administrative support.

This is not a problem that is unique to New York City, or even to the United States. Nor is it a problem unique to physicians, although it is most acute in the medical arena. No country has found a satisfactory means of equalizing the distribution of professionals across its terrain even when compensation is increased or practice location is restricted.

More than any other profession or discipline, it is critical for physicians to be located near their potential patients. Primary care only works if it is easy for people to have access to physicians and this generally means, in the urban context, no more than a few blocks to a physician's office or clinic. Medicaid managed care could conceivably alter the locational dynamic somewhat by reimbursing physicians at a rate that is equal to or possibly even higher than the private market. However, even when the financial deterrents are neutralized, other problems will confound the ability to provide the primary care services that are needed.

The basic issue is whether physicians will want to practice in areas where they are different from their patients. The vast majority of Medicaid recipients in New York City are African-American or Latino, the overwhelming majority of physicians are white. Most of the black physicians are from African countries rather than the United States. It is hard to anticipate whether patients, once they realize they have a choice, will opt to be treated by doctors who are ethnically different from them. No less important, it is not likely that many white physicians will want to stay in areas where they serve few white patients. The possibilities of increasing the pool of minority physicians are limited and the nation's efforts thus far have not been impressive. The number of minority students in medical schools is about the same now as it was twenty years ago, less than 10 percent of the total medical school class.

With the growth of managed care, specialists are likely to find that their practices are dwindling and that they have substantial free time. It is already known that 20 percent of the doctors serving as primary care providers in commercial HMOs in New York City have subspecialty certification. Although these doctors may be willing to accept primary care employment in the absence of better opportunities, it is questionable whether they can function satisfactorily as primary care physicians and as gatekeepers, and whether they will be willing to work among a low income population.

In point of fact it may not be efficient for the health system to deploy physicians with years of training in a subspecialty to manage the everyday care of a relatively well population nor can they do a good job without extensive retraining. Given the economics of medical practice, it is unlikely that subspecialists in New York City have ever treated large numbers of poor people other than in an institutional setting. Moreover, they are accustomed to caring for patients at an advanced stage of illness rather than dealing with preventive care issues. It may require a substantial retraining effort to enable these specialists to work well with the Medicaid population in managed care settings.

While the Medicaid managed care program in its present start-up phase is paying the contractors a good rate, over time it is expected to ratchet down its payments to managed care organizations. The current average payment rate is 88 percent of the AAPCC, but enterprises that have been in the program for some time may get as little as 82 percent. If the managed care companies, in turn, deal with declining Medicaid payments by reducing the amount that goes to primary care providers, it may be even more difficult to get doctors to work for the program. These capacity issues, both physical and human, are the most difficult aspects of the Medicaid managed care initiative and cannot be resolved expeditiously to conform with the time frame envisioned by the state. This does not bode well for the future of the program.

The provision of managed care to a low-income population unaccustomed to having individual attention in other than large institutional settings raises still other issues. It is generally recognized that it takes a long educational effort before patients understand how managed care works and are able to utilize the system effectively and efficiently. People who are used to choosing their own doctors and their own hospitals, and who exercise their own discretion in deciding to see a specialist may find it difficult to work within the guidelines of managed care. It will be even more difficult for people who are used to going to an emergency room for all types of care to adapt to this new system that requires them to see a primary care doctor by appointment and to get prior permission for all other treatment.

With a limited number of people and a long time frame, such an educational process would be possible. It will be far more difficult to carry out given the large numbers of people involved and the rapid timetable for their enrollment in managed care. This will be particularly problematic for New York City since almost everyone in the Medicaid program is accustomed to receiving care *ad lib* in emergency rooms and outpatient departments. Attempts to provide this population with community-based primary care services have not always been successful, particularly in situations when patients were referred to an ER because the primary care center was closed for the evening or the weekend. It does not take long for individuals to realize that it is better to go to the ER and wait than to go to the primary care center and then be sent to the ER and wait. If primary care centers are too distant from a person's home or job, and a medical need arises, it is likely that the person will still travel to the nearest source of care rather than follow the guidelines laid out by the managed care plan.

Another issue is the method of selection and enrollment in a managed care company. Allowing the companies to market directly to Medicaid recipients has not worked for several reasons: the companies were overly aggressive in their pursuit of members and overstated what they could deliver (and underdelivered on their promises); some companies chose to bribe potential members with gifts to join their particular plans; and some companies actually engaged in fraud and deceit to acquire new members. As a result, direct marketing by the companies has been prohibited and the city of New York plans to designate a single firm to perform the marketing and recruitment functions for all the licensed managed care organizations that participate in the Medicaid program. Many other cities and states have run into similar problems with enrollment, so it is unlikely that they can be avoided in New York, even with an outside firm handling this function.

The term of the enrollment period is a related issue. Primary care, by definition, assumes a continuous relationship between the provider and the patient. The managed care companies operate on the basis of a capitation payment which covers all of an individual's medical care needs for a fixed period of time. The Medicaid program, on the other hand, is not designed to be a continuous source of medical care payment. The compromise is to commit the individual to a particular managed care company for a fixed period of time, now set at six months. In case of dissatisfaction with the care received, the enrollee does not have the means to seek other services; therefore the prospect that companies could recruit enrollees and fail to provide adequate services but be guaranteed the six-month capitation may be a strong temptation.

The problem of termination from the Medicaid program is a related issue that interferes with the ability to receive (and to provide) high quality primary care services. These are not insurmountable issues except that the numbers of people, the different types of recipients, and the rapidity with which the state would like to implement the program make them difficult to resolve. It is unclear how primary care will be provided to the homeless population, for example, or to a substance abusing population for whom appointments for care seem unrealistic. Similarly, a person who moves from one area of the city to another may be unable to find a new primary care provider, but will still remain locked into the initial managed care company.

One of the most innovative features of the New York State waiver application is the proposal to place "special needs" populations in managed care organizations. The state expects to license a number of special needs plans (SNPs) that will provide all the resources necessary to care for Medicaid beneficiaries with HIV/AIDS as well as those with mental health problems. There are an estimated 100,000 individuals in each of these categories statewide, with the vast majority residing in New York City.

While there have been many case management programs for the HIV/ AIDS population in other states, there have not been any attempts to capitate the care for this particular group. It cannot be overlooked that people who are enrolled in these managed care plans may find themselves left out of clinical trials or denied treatment with expensive drugs given the capitated nature of the system. How to provide primary care for a large group of people who may be concentrated in particular areas of the city, but who will require substantial attention is also a major problem. The transition of people from standard managed care plans to special needs plans is another, in part for reasons of care, in part because of the differences in the capitation expected by a standard managed care company and by a special needs provider.

The special needs providers for the mentally ill also raise policy and administrative questions. To what extent will care be provided on an ambulatory rather than an inpatient basis and what kinds of utilization thresholds and limitations will be imposed? How will the transition from standard managed care to the special needs plan(s) be managed? Although these are not inherently difficult issues, their rapid resolution in the absence of reliable data for such a large, widely distributed population will be problematic.

The biggest issue involving the transition to Medicaid managed care is its impact on current institutional providers of care. It is expected that managed care will reduce hospital utilization by 20 to 30 percent overall. For the New York City Medicaid population, high utilizers of hospital care, the decline may be in the 40 percent range. Moreover, it is likely that, independent of the number of admissions, inpatient length of stay will be substantially reduced. Given the reliance of hospitals on Medicaid revenues, the financial implications of managed care are dire.

Hospital revenues will be decimated, in addition, by the need to offer discounts to managed care companies if they are to obtain any Medicaid business at all. Thus, not only will occupancy rates drop, but hospitals will also receive less revenue per bed. Moreover, this will occur within a hospital rate setting framework that prohibits hospitals from shifting costs onto other payers. The net impact of managed care will be to reduce hospital occupancy, length of stay, overall admissions, and revenues.

Since Medicaid is responsible for 35 percent of the revenues of voluntary hospitals in New York City and 70 percent of revenues in the public hospital system, and provides care to over 1.5 million residents of the city annually, the severity of these losses should not be underestimated.

Hospitals will try to recapture revenues by contracting with managed care companies, but in a buyer's market they are the weaker party. One response the voluntary hospitals have attempted is the formation of their own Medicaid HMO called HealthFirst. This is an equity organization based around twenty hospitals in New York City which uses the medical staff of the hospital as the provider base. If the hospitals can capture most of the patients, the net effects on their bottom lines will be less severe than if the patients select other managed care providers.

Hospitals in New York City are still reeling from cuts in the Medicaid budget instituted by Governor Pataki. In round terms, over $1 billion was withdrawn from the hospital system in the budget for 1995–96 approved by the legislature in May, 1995. Hospitals are also feeling the impact of for-profit managed care which has grown extensively over the past three years and the impending growth of Medicare managed care which is picking up momentum in the New York area. The net result will be the downsizing (if not closure) of many hospitals in the city with adverse consequences for the provision of the range of services encompassed by comprehensive care, cross-subsidization of the uninsured, and the employment of hospital workers. Let us look at these consequences in greater detail.

There is little question that New York City has been sheltered from the transformations that have affected the nation's health care system over the last decade. New York remained a hospital-centered bastion of academic medical centers and fee-for-service health care delivery within the confines of a regulatory system that set hospital rates and provided for GME and the care of the uninsured. With the growth of managed care, New York is beginning to change as well. Hospitals are closing beds and reducing staff, and the percentage of hospital revenues derived from managed care (now over 15 percent) is increasing. According to the most recent count, the number of New York City residents enrolled in managed care plans (for-profit and Medicaid) is over 1.3 million and continues to grow. The conversion of the Medicaid program to compulsory managed care will more than double this total in a relatively short period. Clearly, the mode of health care delivery in New York City is changing rapidly and the impacts of that change are being felt particularly hard by hospitals.

Most New York hospitals able to do so have tried to become part of networks or systems that include other hospitals and health care entities. The formation of these integrated delivery systems is a means of becoming more attractive to HMOs and also of capturing more health care dollars. The attempts of hospital systems to lower their costs in order to become more competitive and to survive on the discounted rate they must offer the managed care companies have led to the consolidation of services and the closure of units that are not efficient. While these moves may make economic sense from the perspective of the system as a whole, they also make it difficult for people to obtain services that used to be readily available to them. In many cases, what is likely to remain in the community will be an emergency room and a clinic rather than a full-service hospital.

The elaborate mechanisms that are utilized to ensure access for uninsured people are all based on cross-subsidization of their costs that is provided for by NYPHRM. Direct contracting with hospitals by managed care organizations violates the intent of the NYPHRM system (which, paradoxically, allows for it), because it effectively keeps money from getting into the various pools that subsidize care. When HMOs were initially permitted to contract directly with hospitals (in 1988), it was thought that managed care was such a small part of overall revenues that it would have little impact on the system. The experience of the past three years, however, has proved otherwise. With the acceleration of managed care, less money is being collected to repay hospitals for their uncompensated care at the same time that the volume of uncompensated care is increasing. As a result, the ability of hospitals to provide for bad debt and charity care has been eroded.

HMOs argue that since they pay for their members, there is no reason for them to subsidize the costs of nonmembers, an argument that Blue Cross has advanced in the past, and that Medicare continues to advance. HMOs contend that the need to obtain the lowest possible prices in the competitive environment in which they operate means that they cannot afford to make contributions for charity care. What is more, being for the most part for-profit entities, it is not their role to pay for such care. Arguments aside, the impact of these actions is to threaten the continuation of what was in effect universal access to hospital care for residents of New

York City. As the enrollments in managed care organizations grow, the cross-subsidy to care for the poor is becoming a thing of the past.

The other major impact of the growth of managed care on institutions relates to employment. New York has used the Medicare and Medicaid programs to help subsidize the cost of increasing both the size and the wages of the health care workforce. Because health care in New York City is so hospital intensive, a greater proportion of these health workers are employed in hospitals than in other parts of the country. As the move to managed care begins to reduce the need for large hospital capacity, employment is expected to fall as well.

Though inevitable, the contraction of the hospital workforce will have serious consequences for the people whose jobs will be lost and for their relation to the Medicaid program. The vast majority of health workers in New York City hospitals are women, and the vast majority of these women are members of minority groups. Employment in a large institutional setting has meant not only an income and a career ladder, but also health benefits for themselves and their families. As such, hospital employment has kept many people off of the Medicaid rolls.

There would be no problem if there was any assurance that the people who lose their jobs in hospitals would be rehired in new managed care entities, but this is not likely to be the case. For one thing, there is no need in a clinic or managed care setting for most of the jobs performed in hospitals, such as food service, patient transport, and the like. For another, a hospital operates around the clock while ambulatory care tends to be a daytime service requiring many fewer employees. Further, while the hospitals are located in the communities where workers live, offices of the managed care organizations may not be so conveniently reached. Thus there is a real likelihood that one of the results of the growth of Medicaid managed care will be an increase in the welfare and Medicaid rolls with people who formerly were employed by hospitals.

The growth of Medicaid managed care will also have serious consequences for the funding of graduate medical education (GME). As with the bad debt and charity care pools, the NYPHRM system requires payers to fund GME. Medicaid contributes $1 billion per year to GME funds. Under direct contracting by managed care companies with hospitals, this money will no longer be explicitly collected and in the movement to decrease costs it is possible that HMOs will refuse to pay for GME. This too, will have a devastating effect on hospitals in New York, not least on their ability to train more primary care doctors. The state could declare GME to be a "public good" and require HMOs to pay for it (along with other payers), but it is uncertain that this could withstand a legal challenge or that it would allow medical schools and hospitals to run GME programs independently as they have in the past.

Over time all of these issues will undoubtedly be addressed in some fashion. However, because Medicaid managed care would represent such a radical departure in the context of the current provision of care in New York, HCFA as of late spring 1996 has yet to approve the state's waiver proposal. Whatever the outcome of the waiver issue, there is no contesting the growth of managed care and particularly Medicaid managed care in New York.

The literature provides a mixed reading of the success of Medicaid managed care in either lowering health care costs or improving quality of care. No other political entity has attempted to transfer so many people from an institutional source of care to managed care in so short a period. The problems that have been noted indicate clearly that the services for Medicaid recipients will not necessarily be improved, at least in the short run. The problems of the non-Medicaid poor will be heightened by the demise of cross-subsidy and the lack of attention to this large and growing segment of the New York City population.

In conclusion, there is really nothing that can be adduced at present to indicate that this latest strategy in caring for the poor will be any more successful than previous strategies. Although there may be comfort in the large number of states that are adopting a managed care approach, there is little evidence that it will work.

8

Destabilization and Beyond

It is easier to make the case that the provision of health care for the poor of New York is likely to undergo major changes in the near and middle term than to describe the new arrangements needed to insure that the almost 2 million Medicaid eligibles and another 1.5 million uninsured individuals will continue to have access to essential medical care. Since all of the payers—government (federal, state, and local), employers, and households—are seeking to moderate their future outlays for health care, our perspective could justifiably be the likely reductions in access and quality of care that will confront the city's poor in the years ahead. However, that would be a one-sided, dysfunctional stance given the long commitment of New York City to providing health services to the poor, and the lack of historic precedent for broadscale national action to disentitle this population to essential services. On the other hand, it would be flying in the face of the current political mood to ignore the more important destabilizing trends that are underway or that are likely to develop in the period immediately ahead, each of which will affect the access of the city's poor to essential health care services. We will consider first governmental actions at federal, state, and local levels that will almost certainly result in significant changes in the organization, financing, and operation of the medical care available to the poor and the uninsured. We will then look at developments in the nongovernmental arenas that are likely to have similar effects.

Third, and most important, we will identify a number of challenges on the horizon that will help to determine how well (or poorly) the political and medical leadership at city and state levels responds to ensure that the poor of New York continue to obtain essential health care services.

Before we seek to chart a path through the uncertain future, it may be useful to identify the major lessons that can be extracted from the last three decades of concerted efforts aimed at improving the health care of New York City's poor. Since past experiences invariably leave their traces on the present and the immediate future a knowledge of their intent and impact can often suggest the bounds within which future changes must evolve and pursue their course. As noted earlier, Medicare enabled the elderly poor to gain entrance to mainstream U.S. medicine, among other reasons because physicians and hospitals were reimbursed liberally for treating the newly covered group.

The arrangements for the poor below sixty-five years of age were less generous and depended on contributions from the states ranging from 20 to 50 percent of their total outlays for the Medicaid-eligible population. The program was inherently compromised by a serious mismatch between the residential patterns of the poor and the practice locations of most American-trained physicians. In New York State, this mismatch was worsened by the inadequate reimbursement (initially $11, now $13) provided for a routine office visit. Faced with an acute shortage of available primary care physicians, most poor people in need of urgent medical care turned to the emergency rooms and clinics of nearby hospitals.

The HHC hospitals located in low-income neighborhoods assumed responsibility for dealing with the large flows of Medicaid and uninsured patients who sought care at their facilities; they were supplemented by local community hospitals and large teaching hospitals that also served substantial numbers of the poor especially in areas where there was no public hospital to which patients could be referred or transferred.

One of the most persuasive lessons of the city's medical care experience over the last three decades and long before that has been the strong and successful efforts of the voluntary hospital system to avoid becoming directly involved with the public hospitals and other public health care facilities. Although selected major AHCs and teaching hospitals entered into affiliation contracts with the city as early as 1961, the affiliates kept an arm's length distance from any institutional commitment to resolving the health care problems of the large numbers of the poor who used public sector institutions. The corollary for policy formulation in New York's health system is that it has proved next to impossible to move towards integrated planning and operations so long as financing and managerial resources are as sharply divided as they have been between the public and voluntary sectors. The failure of the Piel Commission in the late 1960s to effectuate a regional approach with close integration between the two systems is a potent reminder.

Since the mid-1960s the state of New York has been a key regulator of health affairs throughout its jurisdiction, maintaining tight control over hospital reimbursement rates and many other facets of the organization and financing of health care services not only to the Medicaid population which is its federally mandated responsibility, but also to the rest of the population including those with private health insurance.

While the state of New York, as regulator, has undertaken a great many initiatives, among them obtaining a waiver in the early 1980s from HCFA to operate an all-payer system (Medicare included), it is worth mentioning an old adage of economists—that regulators tend to become captive of those they regulate. In assessing the experience of New York State as regulator, one should be reminded of the sensitivity of various governors to the claims of unionized hospital employees in successive wage conflicts with the hospital sector. On various occasions the state's political leadership persuaded the hospitals to settle for higher wages and improved benefits, promising to take such action into account in revising hospital reimbursement rates.

To cite another instance: When the Hospital Association of New York State (HANYS) calculated in 1985 that the renewal of the HCFA waiver would cost the state about $250 million annually in federal reimbursements, the state legislature was persuaded not to request a renewal. What these and numerous other examples confirm is that in a political democracy with power heavily concentrated among persons of wealth and the higher management ranks of private and nonprofit institutions, public officials are severely constrained in the policies that they can initiate and enforce.

Except in extreme cases, such as the decision of the city of New York in the late 1970s to close Sydenham Hospital in Harlem, it is generally very difficult to organize low-income neighborhoods to protect or expand the limited health care resources to which they have access. For the most part the poor do not have much leverage on local politicians and even less on state and federal elected and appointed officials.

Several other factors relating to the political disenfranchisement of most low-income neighborhoods in New York City should be noted. First, there is the absence of a political voice in the poorest areas because of the flight of the preexisting local leadership as neighborhoods deteriorated. Second, a high proportion of eligible voters fail to register and vote; hence it is that much easier for politicians and legislatures to ignore local concerns. The inflow during the past decade of about a million new immigrants, many or most of whom are too preoccupied with simple survival to become politically active, further contributes to the weakness of low-income neighborhoods to enforce their demands for better health care.

Moreover, New York City, like most political entities, has lacked any independent body, public or private, that is charged with evaluating the effectiveness with which $44 billion of annual health care expenditures are being utilized and pointing directions for improving the health care services available to the city's poor.

Destabilization in the Governmental Arena

While the details, as of early 1996, still remain to be negotiated between Congress and the Clinton administration regarding the scale and timing of reductions in the rate of future federal spending for Medicare and Medicaid as well as for selected health care functions such as graduate medical education (GME), the odds favor significant deceleration in spending for the out-years.

Again, while the details have yet to be worked out between the Republicans and the Democrats as to longer-term constraints on federal spending for Medicare and Medicaid, the odds suggest that Congress may not continue Medicaid as an open-ended entitlement program. Further, Congress is likely to explore and probably enact a number of alternative provisions to encourage Medicare enrollees to opt for a less open-ended fee-for-service benefit structure. The critical point in the context of the potential reduction in the access of the city's poor to essential health care services is that with governmental funds accounting for more than half of the $44 billion current annual outlays, and with the federal government by far the largest of the three governmental contributors to the financing of health care, the prospect of even a modest retardation in the rate of prospective federal spending is a severe threat to the city's poor.

We will look next at the present and prospective decision-making environment of the state along a series of fronts—organization, financing, and operations—of the health care system with a focus on the city's poor. New York has long sponsored a more liberal Medicaid program than any other large state, with average per capita outlays twice those of California. On the other hand, given New York State's severe budgetary pressures, it is inevitable that the governor and the legislature will find ways to moderate future expenditures for health care, the second largest item after appropriations for education.

The vulnerability of the city's poor to present, and more particularly, to prospective cutbacks in spending on medical care is compounded by the fact that with slightly more than 40 percent of the state's total population, New York City accounts for about 65 percent of the state's Medicaid-eligible population and outlays. Upstate legislators will be disinclined to raise additional tax revenue to help shore up the costly health care delivery system for the city's poor.

Even in the absence of geographic tensions one must note that New York State for a variety of reasons, including its traditional liberal support for health care and other social services, finds itself in a trap. Its corporate and personal income tax rates are considerably higher than those prevailing in other states which have thereby become a more hospitable environment for both corporations and wealthy individuals. As a result, New York State has lagged in its recent rate of economic growth.

With many new managed care plans entering the New York City market subsequent to the state's Medicaid-managed care legislation of 1991 and with most of the older plans making strong efforts to expand, the newly elected governor, George Pataki, and his administration decided early in 1995 to accelerate the enrollment of Medicaid eligible individuals in managed care plans. However, within a few months, both local and state officials recognized that the aggressive marketing tactics pursued by many of the managed care plans required reassessment and the enrollment process subjected to greater control and supervision. The plans overpromised on the care they would deliver and underdelivered on the care they provided. What is more the U.S. Department of Health and Human Services was dilatory, if not reluctant, to grant New York State's request for a waiver that would facilitate its efforts to enroll expeditiously most Medicaid eligibles.

As of early 1996, implementation of the Medicaid managed care program is contingent upon the resolution of several issues. First, how long will it take to put in place an improved enrollment process that will meet the requirements of both the responsible state officials and the individuals and families that are being recruited? Second, to what extent will the competing managed care plans succeed in recruiting additional physicians who are willing to practice in neighborhoods readily accessible to most Medicaid eligibles? And third, how difficult will it be for the state of New York to identify and contract with new providers of managed care services for the more complex and problematic subgroups of Medicaid beneficiaries such as the elderly, the disabled and the blind who together account for close to two-thirds of all Medicaid outlays?

All signs point to a reduction in the numbers of the Medicaid-eligible population following the prospective reductions in federal, state, and local financing for the program in 1996 and beyond. This raises the question of how the considerable number of the poor who will be removed from the Medicaid rolls and the large numbers of the uninsured will be able to obtain the basic care that they will need in the months and years ahead.

A closely related question that likewise involves the future direction of state health policy, is what will happen after the expiration of NYPHRM on June 30, 1996? For the better part of three decades, New York State has pursued a strong regulatory approach whose basic mechanism has been tighter control of reimbursement to acute care hospitals and other health care providers. Private payers such as insurance companies and Blue Cross have been assessed a compulsory surcharge on their payments to create a bad debt and charity pool the proceeds of which have been distributed to hospitals in proportion to the amounts of uncompensated care that they provide the poor. Although the Supreme Court ruled unanimously in May, 1995 that the New York State statute was not in violation of ERISA, it is uncertain at present whether the state legislature will perpetuate its policy of hospital rate regulation or decide to give the market broadened scope—possibly even lifting the long-standing ban against the operation in New York State of for-profit hospital chains.

Given these uncertainties about the scope and direction of future state health policy, it is questionable that the regulatory mechanisms that have been directly tied to the financial survival of acute care hospitals with special consideration for those that offer large amounts of care to the poor will continue to be the primary axis of state action. The probability of a major shift in goals and mechanisms is increased once account is taken of the surplus of acute care hospital beds in most regions in the state. The state officialdom is more likely to direct its regulatory powers to the elimination of excess beds rather than perpetuate its earlier strategy which was primarily directed to enabling hospitals at financial risk to continue serving the local poor.

We will now turn to the third level of government—the government of New York City—to assess the challenges that it faces on the health care front and the range of its possible responses. Shortly after his election in November 1994, Mayor Rudolph Giuliani, confronting a serious structural budget deficit, declared that the time had come for New York City to withdraw from the direct provision of health care services and proposed the lease or sale of the eleven acute care hospitals and other health care facilities that comprise the Health and Hospitals Corporation (HHC). However, the mayor made it clear, particularly in his response to the report of his *Advisory Panel on the Future of the Health and Hospitals Corporation* (August 1995) that the city did not plan to abandon the poor and the uninsured, leaving them to find and pay for medical care however they could. His only intent was that the city government should no longer be the direct provider of health care services.

The executive director of the Mayoral Advisory Panel, Maria K. Mitchell, special advisor to the mayor for health policy and chair of the Health and Hospitals Corporation, together with the six other members of the Panel made the following recommendations in their report:

- the mayor should establish a committee to speed the dissolution of HHC, with the city continuing to help finance the health care of the poor which would be provided by the nongovernmental sector;
- the decentralization of HHC should be accelerated to facilitate removing the city from the ownership and operation of health delivery systems;
- a review of options for each facility and provider agency currently under HHC;
- the formation of a taskforce on worker training;
- the creation of an independent panel to monitor quality of care.

In support of these and other recommendations, the panel emphasized the vulnerability of the HHC system in an era of expanding managed care; the disproportionate amounts of public funds that are directed to health care in New York City compared to other large cities; the need to eliminate about 10,000 hospital beds in New York City in the foreseeable future; and the urgent necessity to provide more and better primary and preventive care to most of the poor rather than episodic hospital-based care, ambulatory and inpatient.

The panel estimated that the city contributed a total of $4.2 billion to health care services for Medicaid beneficiaries ($2.4 billion) and the uninsured ($1.8 billion) during 1994. The context for these expenditures should be noted. Total expenditures for health care in New York City in 1994 are estimated to be $44 billion; the combined contributions of the federal, state and local governments to this total come to about $23 billion. In light of likely future trends in government funding, the vulnerability of Medicaid's share—over 21 percent—is obvious.

There are other dimensions of health care financing and delivery in New York City that must also be factored into alternative forecasts of the care that will be available to the city's poor in the future. Not to be overlooked is the differentially large role of the city's academic health centers in the operation of graduate medical education and the role that the residents in these programs play in caring for the poor. We will also have to consider briefly the extent to which geography and socioeconomic characteristics have resulted in a bifurcated health care delivery system, one for the insured middle class and the affluent and the other for the poor. And finally we must consider the growing conviction among the medical leadership that the major challenge facing the city's poor is the ability to obtain comprehensive primary care services in their community.

Before we look more closely at the opportunities—present or potential—to ensure access for the poor to essential care in a period of more constrained health care spending, we should consider the disproportionate number of residents, among them a very large subset of international medical graduates (IMGs), who are enrolled in GME programs. Although New York City accounts for less than 3 percent of the nation's total population its hospitals currently provide training to about 11,000 residents of a national total of some 100,000. IMGs constitute over 50 percent of all hospital residents in New York City.

A number of discrete but interconnected aspects of GME are likely to have significant impact on the future mission and financing of the major teaching hospitals in New York City as well as on the delivery of health care services to the poor and the uninsured. Most informed observers believe that Congress will reduce significantly the amount of funding, currently in the $5 to $6 billion range, that Medicare has been providing to help underwrite GME. It is less clear whether Congress will, at the same time, also decide to reduce the number of IMGs who are accepted into accredited GME programs from the present figure of about 35 percent of the annual number of U.S. medical school graduates to as low as 10 percent, a measure that many of the leaders of American medical education recommend.

New York State, as part of its regulatory apparatus, has not depended solely on Medicare to support GME training. It has also required Blue

Cross and other private sector payers to contribute to the total pool of available dollars so that teaching hospitals in the city currently receive about $200,000 per annum for each resident in an accredited program. Clearly, a significant reduction in Medicare funding for GME and a parallel cutback in the number of IMGs who can be reimbursed with Medicare dollars would have serious disruptive effects for the future operation of the large teaching hospitals in New York City in terms both of their revenue flows and of the new cost pressures that they would face as they replaced residents with other medical personnel, ranging from board certified physicians to nurses and physician assistants. From an operational perspective the most exposed hospitals would be those in the HHC system. Except for two hospitals that share integrated residency programs with their affiliates, IMGs currently account for the great majority of HHC residents, ranging from 62 percent to 84 percent. In the face of the extreme vulnerability of public hospitals in New York City and in selected other locations where they provide much of the hospital-based care to the poor, federal legislation should be aimed at a phased schedule of cutbacks.

What are the issues relating to financing and operations that face the nongovernmental health sector, in the first instance, the not-for-profit acute care hospitals; the managed care companies, by and large for-profit; and the large number of physicians in private practice, over 25,000, most of whom are specialists with only a minority practicing a primary care discipline?

There are two ways to approach the nongovernmental institutions and entities. One is to focus on selected changes in their circumstances and the actions which some have taken to respond to the challenges that the rapidly changing environment has presented. A second is to look at some of the changes, now under way and impending, to which key players are in an early adaptive phase, at the same time that others are trying to comprehend what lies ahead in order to develop a meaningful strategy.

The seven academic health centers (AHCs) and their major teaching hospitals have become increasingly aware during the past few years that they could not depend upon the approaches that had served them for most of the three decades since the passage of Medicare and Medicaid. Despite rigid state control over the number of authorized hospital beds, New York City faces a surplus estimated by the Mayor's Advisory Panel at 10,000 out of a current total of 35,000 beds. Compared to most other large urban centers, length of patient stay in New York City hospitals is well above average. Moreover, until recently enrollment in managed care plans has had desultory growth; the recent spurt and anticipated expansion in the next few years point to much reduced inpatient utilization in the future. Several recent building projects, such as the Milstein Hospital Building at Presbyterian Hospital, overshot the market. It is probably no exaggeration to say that each of the seven AHCs has more beds than it currently needs and certainly will need in the future as demand heads sharply downward.

Faced with the threat of underutilized inpatient capacity, most of the AHCs have adopted one or another variant of networking that seeks to tie outlying community hospitals, mostly in the other boroughs and in the suburbs, into an evolving system in which the academic health center's professional and technological strengths are made selectively accessible to the new members of the network in return for referrals of patients requiring tertiary or quaternary care to the AHC. The terms of the quid pro quo are many and complex, but the critical question is whether the volume of new patient referrals to the AHCs will enable them to meet their revenue and teaching targets. It will require a number of years of experimentation before it is known whether any of the current networking efforts will prove successful. However, it is highly unlikely that these efforts will ensure the survival of all seven AHCs.

A second reason for the current and future vulnerability of the AHCs is the fact that during the past two decades all of them have vastly expanded their faculties with clinicians who spend most of their time treating private patients. These clinicians make important contributions from their earnings to their departments as well as to the dean's fund to help finance special projects. Despite the relatively slow growth until recently in managed care enrollments in the city, the proportion of insured patients who now belong to such plans, about 20 percent, is of a magnitude that threatens the future revenues of the AHCs. Far fewer managed care enrollees are admitted for inpatient treatment; most managed care plans tend to restrict the access of enrollees to specialists; and managed care plans seek increasingly to contract with hospitals and physicians that are willing to offer them price-sensitive rates and/or capitation.

While most of these anticipated changes lie in the future, only an unreconstructed optimist would deny that they will become more and more common. Because of present and potential gaps between revenues and expenditures, a growing number of AHCs and their principal teaching affiliates began some years ago to take a hard look at the expense side of their ledgers with an aim of reducing their outlays. Many leading hospitals have sought to diminish substantially their cadres of middle and upper managers; others have examined their nursing patterns and replaced fair numbers of high earning nurses (with salaries of $65,000 and above) with larger cadres of recent graduates. Almost all hospitals, those with strong as well as those with weak balance sheets, are reexamining their capital investments to be sure that they have urgent need for proposed new, costly equipment and improved or expanded facilities. And there are numerous other cost-saving approaches that many are considering, have launched, or are implementing.

Withal, a major challenge remains. The dominance of the hospital as the center of the U.S. health care system—a position that it has held since the end of World War II—is clearly drawing to an end. In its place will be an integrated healthcare network in which hospitals will continue to play an important role but more at the periphery than at the center. The impact and implications of this major reconfiguration cannot be actually described and assessed before it materializes and that is still some time off—at least in New York City. It is possible that if the Mayoral Panel recommendations are implemented, not only by the city but also by voluntary sector institutions, the process of transforming the free-standing hospital into an integrated network will accelerate. But, as is noted below, most of the city's AHCs and major teaching hospitals will be able to venture seriously into such a transformation only if political leaders, hospital trustees, and medical leaders develop the structure and the financing that will be needed for successful integration.

It is evident that the near and middle term will be characterized nationally and locally by increasing destabilization of the dominant acute care hospital-centered system of the past third of the century. As far as New York City is concerned—and more particularly the provision of health care services to the poor and the uninsured—the state Department of Health has been advocating for at least a decade a shift in strategy aimed at the establishment and expansion of community-based clinics. In the late 1980s, the HHC recognized the logic of this approach and took at least initial steps to implement it programmatically. More recently, the city in cooperation with the state has initiated actions aimed at the same goal and is eliciting the assistance of not-for-profit groups that are able to sponsor and direct new or expanded community health clinics.

Any serious effort to improve the health care of the New York City poor should build on earlier, acknowledged but only partially realized goals involving expanded and improved ambulatory care services. Defining the target of opportunity is a necessary step in the pursuit of effective health care services for the city's poor but it is only a first step. The critical concomitant issues are the identification of the interested parties that must play a role in the effort together with the actions that key players in the governmental and voluntary sectors must engage in to realize the potential of improved ambulatory care for the poor.

Before we examine the potential of an expanded and strengthened effort focussed on community-based health clinics it may be helpful to summarize some key aspects of the current destabilization trends that have direct bearing on such a program in the years ahead. Without ascribing any special significance to their order, the points recapitulated below help to frame the approach that we have identified:

- In the face of universal pressures to constrain the growth of future outlays for health care services, the only prospect for improving ambulatory care services for the city's poor would be through the redeployment of "excess" resources that are underutilized in the delivery of existing health care services. To illustrate: In many low-income areas of the city, about one in six patients treated in the emergency room of an HHC hospital is admitted to the hospital for what is termed an ASC (ambulatory sensitive condition), meaning that with timely and appropriate access to primary care services the inpatient admission could have been avoided. There is clearly significant potential for improving ambulatory care services for the poor if such a resource redistribution could be carried through.
- A related opportunity for resource redistribution: The Mayoral Panel of August 1995 suggested that New York City could reduce its inpatient capacity, both in the municipal and voluntary sector, by some 10,000 out of a current total of 35,000 certified acute care beds. With the level of acute care hospital expenditures now approximating $20 billion yearly, a reduction of almost 30 percent of inpatient capacity could translate into a potential release of billions of dollars of resources. If only partially realized and redeployed, this sum would be more than ample for a substantial expansion and improvement of ambulatory care facilities for the poor.
- The desire, in fact the determination, of Mayor Giuliani to get the HHC out of the direct delivery of health services, particularly inpatient care, will not be easy to implement for a variety of reasons, chiefly the threat that it would represent to the health care of the neighborhood poor. Most HHC

hospitals in low-income areas are "essential community providers," which means that if the hospital closes its doors the poor are likely to be left with no ready source of essential medical care.

- In many low-income neighborhoods the HHC hospital is the dominant economic enterprise providing more jobs and more income than any other local activity. If the convertible sections of these local hospitals were remodeled to provide expanded and improved ambulatory care services for the residents of the community, several barriers that currently stand in the way of the mayor's plan would be lowered, if not removed. The new facility would continue to serve as a major health resource for the local community. A significant number of jobs and income previously generated by the hospital would continue to be available to the local population. And there would be an opportunity to upgrade the quality of the ambulatory care services for the community if one or another prestigious teaching hospital would assume responsibility for defining and monitoring professional standards in association with selected community leaders.
- The Mayoral Advisory Panel and its predecessor, the Barondess Commission (1992), pointed out the need to strengthen the quality of ambulatory care services that the HHC clinics and emergency rooms provide. The waiting time for an initial appointment at many of the clinics is excessive; most patients never see the same physician on successive visits; physicians are unable to retrieve patient records when they must decide on diagnostic and therapeutic measures; there is no effective outreach to patients suffering from one or more chronic diseases. All of these speak to the opportunities for improving the quality of ambulatory care via expanded and improved community health clinics. With the effective redeployment of resources now devoted to inpatient care, considerable numbers of local residents could be hired and trained as health outreach workers.

There is little reason for serious concern about the ability and willingness of the voluntary institutions to provide inpatient care for the Medicaid eligible population. Most voluntary hospitals welcome the opportunity to admit Medicaid patients, attested by the fact that in recent years their revenue from Medicaid has exceeded all other payments for inpatient care. Facing a decline in admissions, shortened length of stay, and excess bed capacity it is a safe presumption that the voluntary sector—assuming continuation of current reimbursement levels—will not hesitate to take responsibility for inpatient care for the entire Medicaid population, given time to make the necessary adjustments in areas where such admissions might increase precipitously.

The more complicated challenge relates to the ability and willingness of the voluntary hospitals to treat the sizable numbers of uninsured patients who are currently cared for in HHC hospitals. Here several issues are critical. First, Mayor Giuliani has stated repeatedly that his aim to terminate direct delivery of health care services by the HHS does not imply that the city will abandon its historic commitment to provide all persons access to essential care irrespective of their ability to pay. Hence the city would have to establish, actually reestablish, a system of reimbursing voluntary hospitals for providing care to the low-income uninsured.

A second consideration is the action that the state of New York will take to address the problem of bad debt and charity expenditures when the current reimbursement mechanism, NYPHRM, expires at the end of June 1996. Closely related is the policy that the federal government will pursue with respect to future appropriations for "disproportionate share" payments to hospitals that provide large amounts of unreimbursed care.

It appears likely that prospective payments by the federal government to such hospitals will be significantly reduced but, given the increasing numbers of uninsured persons, the total elimination of disproportionate share payments is unlikely. The challenge to the city of New York would be to work out an arrangement with the state that would channel state funds for the care of the city's poor to the city government for suballocation to the principal providers. If at all possible, the city of New York should explore the possibility of directing the federal disproportionate share payments similarly, first to the city and through the city to the providers of services to the poor.

Even if substantial progress could be achieved in freeing up many of the earmarked dollars that currently go to support excess inpatient capacity in the HHC and the voluntary hospital sector and greater discretion was yielded to the city to use special payments from the state and the federal governments to expand ambulatory care services to the poor, it is still questionable whether Mayor Giuliani's aim to terminate direct health care delivery by the HHC has much prospect of near- or mid-term success. As we have suggested, a precondition for such action would be the continued operation of substantial health care services in locations where HHC currently provides not only medical care but also jobs and income to the local population.

Assuming that the city would be able to elicit the cooperation of most low-income neighborhoods to such a conversion, could the leadership of nearby AHCs or major teaching hospitals be persuaded to assume responsibility for former HHC hospitals that will be in the process of transition to major community health care clinics? While there is no a priori answer to this question, the weight of the evidence suggests that such a change should be feasible. In the first instance one can point to the fact that all seven AHCs that operate residency training programs in the city have been involved both professionally and financially in assisting the HHC hospitals in caring for the local poor.

One must also recall that the HHC has been allocating about a half-billion dollars annually to underwrite their affiliation contracts. At the same time, the seven AHCs that sponsor graduate medical education programs in the five boroughs are involved in varying degrees with low-income communities, from Einstein-Montefiore at one end of the spectrum to Cornell-New York Hospital at the other.

We have mentioned the growing dependence of these major institutions on their Medicaid revenues which are likely to be of increasing importance in the future. We have also noted the potentiality for the city of New York to combine some of its own outlays with state and federal revenues to underwrite at least in part, the costs of treating the uninsured and this, in turn, should be an incentive for the AHCs and their principal teaching affiliates to assume a new leadership role in directing quality community clinics. Not to be ignored is the threat that the city of New York might reduce drastically the half-billion dollars of revenue that it contributes annually to the academic health centers with which it has affiliation agreements.

Over and above current and prospective market and political changes, one must consider the changing educational missions of the AHCs. The era of virtually exclusive preoccupation with the training of specialists in a hospital environment is coming to a close. No medical school or major teaching hospital can afford not to educate tomorrow's physicians in ambulatory care settings and in the process to become increasingly engaged in health education, preventive services and health status. In short, what the poor most need—improved access to readily accessible, enhanced ambulatory care services—is the counterpart of what the AHCs most need today and tomorrow—the opportunity for their staff and students to practice medicine and perform research in ambulatory care settings far more extensively than they have. In marked contrast to the last three decades during which the medical leadership was preoccupied with hospital-based training and patient care, the era ahead suggests that ambulatory care, community partnerships, and the health of the public will become the preferred orientation of both AHCs and their low-income neighbors.

Some researchers, informed by New York State's mandatory program of Medicaid managed care enrollment, will argue that the preceding emphasis on expanded ambulatory care centers under the professional leadership of AHCs and leading teaching hospitals working collaboratively with local community leaders is misdirected if not counterindicated. We disagree. Our skepticism regarding the potential of managed care to provide more and better health care for neighborhoods with large concentrations of poor persons is based on professional, political and economic factors. For the better part of the last half century, graduates of U.S. medical schools have avoided setting up private practices in low-income neighborhoods and there is little if any evidence that they are about to change. In the absence of a reversal in physician preferences and behavior it is difficult to imagine how Medicaid managed care based on an IPA model is likely to grow rapidly and to provide a higher level of care for the poor. Moreover, about two-thirds of all Medicaid outlays go for special categories of patients such as the seriously disabled, a group with which most managed care systems have had little experience and usually seek to avoid.

There is another lesson from the post-World War II experience in the delivery of health care services in New York City that warrants attention. Most physicians in private practice have avoided accepting Medicaid patients not only because of the low reimbursement rates but also because of their concern that most of their private patients do not wish to mingle in the waiting room with persons on welfare. While the reimbursement rates for physicians must be increased if the poor and the uninsured are to gain access to a better and more comprehensive level of ambulatory care—as the state of New York has provided in selected demonstration programs—the odds favor the continuation of a bifurcated ambulatory health care delivery system, one for persons in low-income neighborhoods the other for those living in middle-class neighborhoods.

An appreciable number of New Yorkers view the continuation of a bifurcated health care delivery system as undemocratic, inequitable and even unjust. Admitted. Nevertheless, it is important to remember that when the American people and the Congress were put to the test by the Clinton health reform proposals in 1994, considerations of justice and equity in the future financing and delivery of health care were given short shrift. This is not to say that the American public may not decide some years hence to reverse this position and opt for a single standard of governmentally financed health care services for all. But given the vast differentials that continue to prevail in the U.S. with respect to income, housing, education and other critically important services, it would be unrealistic in the extreme to ignore the potential of expanding and improving ambulatory care services for the poor on the ground that this action left them short, even far short, of the health care services available to the affluent.

9

Lessons for Policy

The principal justification for an in-depth study such as this, which has probed the experiences of the last three decades during which massive funding became available to improve the health care of the nation—and more specifically the health care of the New York City poor—is to extract lessons that can help to guide policy in the future, aware that the future will be marked by wide-reaching change.

Accordingly, this chapter will first identify the most important policy lessons that we have been able to distill from our three decade review and analysis; and second, will suggest the implications of these lessons for the actions that need to be initiated and implemented in the years ahead if the health care of the poor is to be protected—and improved—in the more constrained financial environment that is imminent.

Lesson 1: Lots of new money can result in the provision of more and better services to the poor. The outstanding case in point are the poor elderly who, because of Medicare, were able to join the mainstream delivery system. Many of the nonelderly poor also gained broader access to both public and voluntary hospitals and clinics and later to nursing homes and home care programs. Moreover, the additional funding made it possible for both the private and public sectors to serve new categories of patients such as the HIV-infected.

Lesson 2: The financial crisis of 1975 that brought New York City close to bankruptcy and the renewed budgetary difficulties that the city has faced since 1989 prove that even large dedicated streams of health care financing may not be able to maintain, much less improve, medical care for the poor. As a result of severe financial pressures, the city has been unable to maintain its capital plant, including its public hospitals, and has lacked adequate and sustained funding needed for preferred delivery systems such as comprehensive community health care clinics. In fact, in response to its fiscal crisis of 1975, the city reduced the scale and scope of its Department of Health to the distinct detriment of the health of the poor: its school health programs were emasculated and its public health monitoring activities curtailed, thereby facilitating the proliferation of new drug-resistant strains of tuberculosis. As the foregoing illustrations indicate, improving the health care of the poor requires the city to have access to capital to maintain (and preferably enhance) its health care facilities and its capability to conduct a strong public health effort. Maintaining, even expanding, access to ambulatory and inpatient care, is not sufficient.

Lesson 3: The problems that the Health and Hospitals Corporation has faced in managing its eleven acute care hospitals and other facilities is a potent reminder of the inherent difficulties of operating a large municipal health care system efficiently and effectively, especially if the more influential sectors of the electorate do not utilize the public institutions.

It took the city over fifteen years to reorganize its billing system to enable it to collect payments due it from Medicare, Medicaid and private insurance companies. The city was never able to recruit and retain the cadre of competent health care administrators that it needed to manage its eleven hospitals, partly because its salaries were not competitive and partly because it was unable and unwilling to delegate adequate authority to its hospital managers. The operation of the sizable municipal health care sector was further complicated by the fact that local politicians saw the local hospital as their patronage preserve and the mayor had to negotiate with a powerful union that had political as well as economic muscle. Moreover, the relationships between the central HHC board and staff and the individual hospitals were strained throughout these years.

Lesson 4: The voluntary hospitals which have long dominated the New York City acute care sector continued their historic tradition of providing ambulatory and inpatient care to significant numbers of poor persons after the passage of Medicare and Medicaid. In fact, they attracted the great majority of the poor elderly who were newly covered by Medicare. They also continued to provide considerable inpatient care for the Medicaid population, accounting in 1995 for the majority of Medicaid hospital admissions. Their emergency rooms and clinics served considerable numbers of Medicaid patients as well. True, the voluntary institutions were reluctant initially to treat patients suffering from AIDS but when pressed by the state commissioner of health they responded, if somewhat reluctantly. The only group of patients that the voluntary hospitals sought to deflect to the public hospitals were the uninsured for whom neither the state nor the city provided direct reimbursement.

What is striking is that New York City has operated two parallel systems of hospital and ambulatory care for many decades without any serious efforts at coordination. In fact, the aftermath of the Piel Commission report in the late 1960s which recommended greater collaboration, if not outright integration, of the two sectors was the determination of the voluntary hospitals to avoid establishing closer ties for fear that such action would jeopardize their ability to finance their priority goals specifically education and research alongside patient care.

Lesson 5: It is important to emphasize that despite this arm's length relationship between the voluntary and the public sector institutions, the early 1960s saw the beginning of a special relationship subsumed under the term "affiliation contracts" whereby all but one of the local academic health centers entered into agreements with selected public hospitals to provide them with residents and supervisory medical staff that they were no longer able to recruit themselves. As the white working-class population relocated after World War II to the suburbs, followed by their local practitioners, and younger doctors were unwilling to practice in what became ever more deteriorating neighborhoods, the public hospitals were depleted of professional staff to the point of disaccreditation.

Had it not been for the affiliation contracts that carried an initial price tag of under $2 million rising to $500 million by the mid-1990s, it is difficult to conceive how the HHC could have staffed most of its facilities. Admittedly, the affiliation contracts have been a source of tension between both parties—the city claiming that the medical schools failed to provide adequate professional supervision and the medical schools in turn claiming that the city did not deliver on many of its commitments to improve its hospitals' infrastructures and personnel. Mutual complaints and recriminations notwithstanding, the affiliation contracts became the critical lifeline for the HHC hospitals enabling them to meet their responsibilities for continuing to provide a large proportion of the medical care rendered the city's poor.

Lesson 6: As noted above, the inability of low-income neighborhoods to attract replacements for local practitioners who had relocated or retired created a void for the Medicaid and uninsured population in need of medical care. The graduates of U.S. medical schools had too many desirable alternatives to start practices in areas with large numbers of native-born or immigrant poor, many of them belonging to ethnic or racial minorities. They were further discouraged by the ridiculously low reimbursement rate that the state of New York provided for a routine office visit, $11 and latterly $13. The only opportunities that the residents in these areas had to obtain care from private physicians were from international medical graduates (IMGs) many of whom practiced as members of a "mill" that had learned to game the Medicaid system so that they could earn a living if not flourish.

Although all levels of government made some efforts to subsidize the establishment of private practices in physician shortage areas, none of these efforts was sufficiently strong and/or persistent to overcome the friction of the marketplace. In some impoverished inner city areas there was one private practitioner for 10,000 residents as opposed to one per 500 in an affluent neighborhood. No serious effort to improve the health care of the urban poor can afford to continue to be as remiss as we have been about counteracting the influence of market forces in the locational distribution of physicians.

Lesson 7: Although the public and voluntary hospital systems in New York City have operated in parallel throughout the last three decades, intersecting only in the affiliation program, attention must be focused on the role of the state of New York in the affairs of both systems by virtue of the CON process, the scale and scope of the Medicaid program, reimbursement policies set by successive revisions of NYPHRM, and a host of other levers that the state commissioner of health and the members of his staff were able to exercise. Their influence was reinforced by their ability (demonstrated frequently) to persuade the state legislature to authorize certain new lines of action and to provide additional funding to speed their implementation.

It would, of course, be misleading to infer that Commissioner David Axelrod always got his way in New York City. What is noteworthy, however, is that during his administration, in the 1980s, he was able to exercise strong leadership that kept financially strapped hospitals in low-income areas functioning with the help of special state funds; he was able to bargain with the New York City academic health centers that sought CONs for large expansion and rebuilding programs to make some concessions that expanded opportunities for the neighboring poor to obtain improved access and treatment; he saw to it that the voluntary hospitals shared the burden of treating AIDS patients; and he leveraged the extant dual system so that it became somewhat more responsive to the city's poor. Under Axelrod, the state played a key role in shaping and reshaping the delivery of health care to the city's poor even though its influence was severely limited by the continued existence of the dual (public/voluntary) system.

Lesson 8: With the advantage of lengthened perspective, it is apparent that the health commissioner and Albany had only limited success in bringing about significant changes in the ways in which governmental funds were utilized to support graduate medical education and in modifying the licensing provisions for mid-level medical personnel, particularly nurses, to enlarge their scope of practice.

The state health commissioner made strenuous efforts to persuade the New York City academic health centers to correct what he and his advisors considered a faulty overemphasis on the training of subspecialists at the expense of generalist production. But for the most part the academic health centers refused until quite recently to budge.

On the licensing front, the organized physician community obstructed all but minor concessions to nurses and other mid-level health professionals when it came to broadening the practice codes for nonphysician personnel. It is now obvious that broad action on this front is a sine qua non for any serious efforts to improve the delivery of health care to the inner-city poor, in light of the "avoidance syndrome" that has kept U.S.-trained physicians from practicing in poor communities. Moreover, greater reliance on the utilization of nonphysician personnel as members of medical teams holds promise both of making scarce dollars go further and of providing a range of critical services, such as improved care for the homebound, that physicians tend to ignore.

Lesson 9: One of the more striking reforms that the state legislature has to its credit was legislation in the early 1980s enabling New York City and other municipalities to explore alternatives to costly nursing home care for the increasing disabled and elderly population. So long as Medicaid patients could be cared for at home at no more than 75 percent of the costs incurred at a nursing home, the municipality could authorize treatment at home. New York City, taking advantage of this provision, has developed by far the largest Medicaid home care program in the nation, with more than 60,000 on its rolls. This program was, in fact, so popular that the state legislature placed a ceiling some years ago on further expansion.

Lesson 10: The state legislature must also be credited with taking action in the mid-1980s to reassess its long-term ban on licensing for-profit health care providers, which had previously prohibited for-profit managed care companies and for-profit hospital chains from operating in New York State. Recognizing that managed care was proliferating rapidly in other states under the leadership of for-profit companies, the state legislature ended their previous exclusion. The significant growth in HMO enrollments in New York City and New York State after the rescission of the ban on for-profit managed care companies attests to the legislature's reading of the national trend.

At the same time the legislature was not persuaded to revoke the ban on the entrance of for-profit hospital chains into the state. However given the victory of a Republican governor, George Pataki, with his preference for market solutions, the issue is likely to reemerge in the legislative session of 1996.

Lesson 11: Although the state commissioner of health repeatedly urged the academic health centers in New York City to expand the quantity and quality of ambulatory care services that they provided to the city's poor by establishing comprehensive community health care centers in low-income neighborhoods, his message was for the most part unheeded. The leadership of the AHCs had more urgent issues to cope with, particularly the need to increase their sources of funding from practice plan activities as the contribution of government funding dropped from around 70 percent of their budgets in the latter 1960s to under 40 percent in the last decade.

The AHCs appointed large numbers of clinical professors to their faculties to provide ambulatory and inpatient care to an increasing clientele of well insured patients with an understanding that the new appointees would not only cover their own salaries but would also contribute to the budgets of their departments and to the dean's fund. This revenue generating device enabled the AHCs to maintain their educational and research missions and at the same time ensure their continuing financial viability. Most of the AHCs believed that they were discharging their responsibilities to the city's poor by providing a large number of indigent patients with good ambulatory and inpatient care and they did not want to complicate their difficult agendas by responding to the commissioner's challenge.

Lesson 12: There was relatively little energy or money available for innovation during the last decade as the HHC system confronted the need to provide care to increasing numbers of poor persons including new categorical groups such as AIDS patients, the mentally ill, drug addicts, patients infected with new strains of tuberculosis and still others. Further, a large wave of recent immigrants, many neither English-speaking nor covered by insurance, intensified the demands for care on the HHC system.

At the same time, the voluntary sector was forced to look for new ways to increase its revenue flows to maintain its multiple missions of education, research, and top-of-the-line patient care with its insatiable demands for costly technology and a larger more skilled workforce. There was the further need to raise significant new sums to pay for major capital expansions that were underway or had recently been completed.

The parallel health care systems did their best to meet the most urgent needs of the poor but had neither the impetus nor the resources to address the important question of reforming the extant system in the interest of improving the health status of the poor.

Health care analysts and community activists periodically called attention to such ominous trends as the widening gap between various groups of the poor and the citizenry at large in such critical dimensions as infant mortality and average longevity. However, the responsible medical leadership was preoccupied with keeping their respective institutions and systems solvent and responsive to current needs, with limited if any capacity to address opportunities for the extant system to become more responsive to the poor.

Lesson 13: The continuing large-scale absorption within New York City of low-income immigrants, many of whom either were not eligible to vote or simply failed to do so, left many impoverished communities void of the leadership and political following needed to marshal some of the local resources that might make a significant contribution to improving the health care and health status of the local population. Churches, schools, tenant associations, social welfare agencies working together might have had a singular effect by assisting parents to have their children vaccinated or helping to educate the chronically ill to adopt better dietary and physical exercise habits. But without assistance from outside, low-income communities are hard pressed to launch and carry out such self-help efforts.

Lesson 14: It could be said that the single most important insight to be extracted from our historical analysis is the fact that there was no agency in the public or voluntary sector with responsibility for monitoring the dollars that were flowing into New York City to improve the health of the entire citizenry—and more particularly the rapidly growing numbers of its poor. Our calculations of the estimated total expenditures for all health care activities in New York City in 1995 (approximately $44 billion or over $5800 per capita) and the sources of these dollars (about $24 billion from the federal, state and local governments) should have been information routinely available to the public and to the media. An uninformed or poorly informed public cannot be expected to explore opportunities and methods of obtaining for themselves more societal benefits from the resources that are available. Even if the information were available, the interest and the effort to use the information to improve public policy might not be forthcoming. But if no institution in a democratic society is charged with being accountable, then the odds all but rule out the debate, planning, and action required for the citizenry to exploit more effectively the resources potentially at its command. We may, however, soon find ourselves in a period in which resources will be more constrained and the best, probably the only, prospect of meeting the critical needs of the poor and the near-poor is for all interested and concerned parties to become better informed so that they can mount a joint effort to optimize the resources that will be available.

Lesson 15: The final lesson to be drawn is the growing mismatch between the type of ambulatory care available to most of the city's poor and the care that would meet their real needs. At present, the poor obtain primarily episodic care in the emergency rooms and clinics of public or voluntary hospitals, often by physicians who are seeing them for the first time and who have difficulty communicating because of language barriers. Inability to retrieve the patient's previous health record impedes the physician in determining an appropriate treatment plan and results in needless duplication of diagnostic procedures. Comprehensive health care that can enhance the individual's health requires various health personnel organized as a team to instruct patients in better care of themselves and their children and in the use of related ancillary services in the community. This gap between what is provided and what is needed was identified by the state commissioner of health in the early-mid 1980s. His efforts to persuade the principal concerned parties to begin to rectify these systemic flaws had only modest success but the years ahead may provide the stimulus for greater progress.

The current health care financing and delivery system, as it affects the public and the voluntary sectors, is clearly in the early stages of major transformation. Just consider:

- Mayor Giuliani has stated on numerous occasions that he is committed to getting the city out of the provision of direct health care services as promptly as possible and in the interim he is planning to lease or sell three of the eleven HHC hospitals.
- Although the state-mandated enrollment of Medicaid-eligible persons in managed care plans has been temporarily halted, such efforts are likely to be resumed in the near future and this will further place the HHC hospitals at serious risk from reduced patient admissions and revenues.
- Funding for graduate medical education has been targeted for retrenchment by Congress and there is growing pressure in Washington to reduce by an order of magnitude the number of IMGs whose residency training will be subsidized by the federal government. Such action threatens to paralyze the HHC system which is heavily dependent on IMGs for the provision of much/most of the care that it provides to its patients.
- Admissions for inpatient treatment in most HHC hospitals are steadily declining, a trend that is likely to accelerate when enrollment in Medicaid managed care resumes.

It would be a serious error to assume, however, that the only threat to essential health care for the city's poor derives from the uncertain future of the HHC system. The capacity of the voluntary sector to continue to provide the city's poor its accustomed volume and range of ambulatory and inpatient care is likewise uncertain. To note some of the major threats:

- With an estimated surplus of 10,000 acute care beds (of a total of about 35,000 in both systems) the odds favor the closure, merger, or conversion of a substantial number of voluntary hospitals which in turn will reduce, if not eliminate, their ability to continue their efforts on behalf of the poor.
- Traditionally, voluntary hospitals have engaged in a process of cross-subsidization, using their excess revenues from privately insured patients (about 30 percent over their costs) in order to meet expenditures for services that they provided to the poor free of charge or below cost. The continuing enrollment of privately insured persons in managed care plans which have sharply restricted the referrals of their members to the AHCs for consultation or inpatient treatment is rapidly reducing the revenues hitherto available to the AHCs to subsidize the care of the poor.
- In sum: all levels of government are threatening to curtail their funding for Medicare, Medicaid, and other services that the public and private systems have used to pay for their multiple missions including service delivery to the poor. In the face of this ever more ominous outlook for the future fi-

nancing and delivery of essential services to the poor that is a correlate of the diminishing resources likely to be available for both the public and the voluntary hospital systems, the time may be at hand for a conjoint effort by the two sectors, with the mayor taking a leading role, to explore the potential for joint planning and action to optimize the total available dollars.

As the mayor embarks on the process of terminating direct delivery of health care services by the city, there may be an opportunity to explore and implement the following strategic efforts for the poor if the dominant interests, professional and community, can be persuaded to enter into a joint planning exercise: First, the highest priority need in low-income areas is to expand by an order of magnitude comprehensive community health care centers that would be able to provide continuity and quality of care not only for acute conditions but also effect improvements in health status. Second, a window of opportunity may exist for many, if not all, of the HHC hospitals to work out arrangements with nearby voluntary hospitals to assume responsibility for inpatient care to their former patient population. The economics of inpatient care appears to support such a move.

Once the above arrangements are worked out, the challenge would be for the city to take a leadership role in transforming the former HHC hospital plants into the anchor of a much expanded comprehensive community health care network with a neighboring AHC or major teaching hospital and representatives of the community assuming leadership roles. The voluntary AHCs and teaching hospitals have urgent need for more ambulatory training sites which the new comprehensive community care system could provide. The community would have a high stake in the continued employment, often after retraining, of many of the former HHC employees. Further, a much broadened approach to preventive, rehabilitative, and acute care services could generate selective new employment opportunities for community residents.

Clearly there is nothing easy or straightforward about the transition that has been outlined above. But the financing and delivery system that has sustained the hospital sector for most of the last three decades has little prospect of long-term survival. The time has come for a new approach based on cooperative arrangements between the public and the voluntary sectors that was explored by the Piel Commission in the late 1960s but failed, in the deluge of new funding for health care, to appeal to the key parties. However, in the face of a much more constrained funding environment in the years ahead, such a cooperative undertaking warrants priority consideration. There is little prospect for maintaining, much less improving, the delivery of health care services to those in need unless and until the public and the voluntary sectors work together to put in place a more economical and efficient system of delivering quality ambulatory care services to the city's poor focused on the improvement of their health status.

Selected Bibliography

Urban Health Care and the
New York City Health Care System

Studies by the Eisenhower Center for
the Conservation of Human Resources
(formerly The Conservation of Human Resources Project)

Eli Ginzberg. 1949. *A Pattern for Hospital Care.* New York: Columbia University Press.

Eli Ginzberg and Peter Rogatz. 1961. *Planning for Better Hospital Care.* New York: King's Crown Press, Columbia University.

Eli Ginzberg and the Conservation of Human Resources staff. 1971. *Urban Health Services: The Case of New York.* New York: Columbia University Press.

Eli Ginzberg, Alice M. Yohalem, eds. 1974. *The University Medical Center and the Metropolis.* New York: Josiah Macy, Jr. Foundation.

Edith M. Davis and Michael L. Millman. 1983. *Health Care for the Urban Poor.* Totowa, NJ: Rowman and Allanheld.*

Eli Ginzberg, Warren Balinsky, and Miriam Ostow. 1984. *Home Health Care: Its Role in the Changing Health Services Market.* Totowa, NJ, Rowman and Allanheld.

Eli Ginzberg, Edith M. Davis, and Miriam Ostow. 1985. *Local Health Policy in Action: The Municipal Health Services Program.* Totowa, NJ: Rowman and Allanheld.*

Eli Ginzberg and the Conservation of Human Resources staff. 1986. *From Health Dollars to Health Services: New York City 1965–1985.* Totowa, NJ: Rowman and Allanheld.*

Eli Ginzberg, Howard S. Berliner, and Miriam Ostow. 1993. *Changing U.S. Health Care: A Study of Four Metropolitan Areas.* Boulder, CO: Westview Press.*

---

* Sponsored by the Robert Wood Johnson Foundation.

131

Government Reports

Commission on the Delivery of Personal Health Services (Piel Commission). *Comprehensive Community Health Services for New York City.* December 1967.

The Mayor's Commission on the Future of Child Health. *The Future of Child Health in New York City.* New York City Department of Health, August 1989.

The Mayor's Management Advisory Task Force. *Report on Health Care.* Program Planners, Inc. and the New York City Health Systems Agency, April 1991.

The Mayoral Commission to Review the Health and Hospitals Corporation. *Report.* November 1992.

The Governor's Health Care Advisory Board. *Workforce Needs for a Reforming Health Care System.* December 1994.

Betsy McCaughey, Lieutenant Governor. *Report to Governor George E. Pataki Regarding the State Fiscal Year 1995–1996.* Medicaid Budget. January 18, 1995.

State of New York, Office of the State Comptroller. *Review of the Financial Plan of the City of New York for Fiscal Years 1996 through 1999.* Report 4-96. July 24, 1995.

Mayoral Advisory Panel for the Health and Hospitals Corporation. *Report.* August 1995.

Nongovernment Reports

United Hospital Fund of New York

Melena Hill Walker. *Building Bridges: Community Health Outreach Worker Programs.* July 1994.

Rick Sarpin, Kathryn Haslanger, and Steven Dawson. *Better Jobs, Better Care: Building the Home Care Work Force.* August 1994.

Annual Report, 1994–95.

Melvin I. Krasner. *Monitoring Medicaid Managed Care: Developing an Assessment and Evaluation Program.* 1995.

Community Service Society of New York

Mink Ly Griffin. *Health and Health Care Profile of NYC's New School Applications 1990–1991.* 1993.

Poverty in New York City, 1993, An Update.

Visiting Nurse Service of New York
Annual Report, 1992–93.

Citizens Budget Committee
Political Leadership in the Two New Yorks: Fiscal Policy in the 1990s. June 1993.
Poverty and Public Spending Related to Poverty in New York City. August 1994.
Modernizing the Municipal Employee Health Insurance Program. April 1995.

The Kaiser Commission on the Future of Medicaid
Medicaid and Managed Care: Lessons from the Literature. March 1995.

The Presbyterian Hospital-Columbia Presbyterian Medical Center
Patient Origin Patterns: Inpatients, Ambulatory. April 1982.
Community Health Care: Allen Pavilion, Ambulatory Care Network Corporation, Presbyterian Hospital. May 1995.

Special Studies

Nora Piore, Purlaine Lieberman, and James Linnane. *Health Expenditures in New York City: A Decade of Change.* Columbia University Center for Community Health Systems. 1976.
————. "Public Expenditures and Private Control? Health Care Dilemmas in New York City." *Milbank Memorial Fund Quarterly/Health and Society.* Winter 1977.
Richard Garfield and David Abramson, eds. *Washington Heights/Inwood: The Health of a Community.* The Health of the Public Program at Columbia University. June 1994.
John Billings, et al. "Impact of Socioeconomic Status on Hospital Use in New York City." *Health Affairs.* Spring 1993.
Howard S. Berliner and Susan Nesbitt. *Structural Characteristics of Primary Care Physicians in IPA-Type HMOs in New York City: 1992–1993.* Final Report submitted to the Health Services Improvement Fund. March 1995.
Charles Brecher and Sheila Spiezo. *Privatization and Public Hospitals.* New York: Twentieth Century Fund. 1995.
Crain's New York Business. Health Care, Picking up the Pieces. November 21, 1994.
Crain's New York Business. Health Care. January 23, 1995.

Data Sources

The principal data sources for this study were the ongoing statistical information and special reports produced by the following government and nongovernment agencies:

Index

Academic health centers (AHCs). *See also* Affiliation contracts; Graduate medical education (GME); International medical graduates (IMGs)
  affiliation contracts, 2–3, 117, 123
  biomedical research, 5
  expansionary forces influencing, 15, 57, 126
  graduate medical education (GME), 2, 56, 62–63, 64, 125
  and health care destabilization, 110–19
  and poor, 126, 129–30
  and public hospitals, 2–3, 123–24
Acquired immunodeficiency syndrome (AIDS), 7, 39, 87, 96–97, 127
Administrative management. *See also* Labor unions; Regulation
  governmental, 106–11
  Health and Hospitals Corporation (HHC), 6–7, 8, 37–39, 72–74, 122
  historical analysis of, 122, 127–28, 129–30
  Montefiore Medical Center, 63–64
  nongovernmental, 111–18
  political influences on, 105–11, 114–15, 116, 118–19
  voluntary hospitals, 3, 9, 104
Advisory Panel on the Future of the Health and Hospitals Corporation (1995), 109–10, 111, 113, 114–15
Aetna, 70
Affiliation contracts. *See also* Academic health centers (AHCs); Graduate medical education (GME); International medical graduates (IMGs)
  Academic health centers (AHCs), 2–3, 117, 123

  Health and Hospitals Corporation (HHC), 36, 37, 111, 117, 123
  public hospitals, 2–3, 35–36, 117, 123
  voluntary hospitals, 2–3, 117, 123
Aid to Families with Dependent Children (AFDC), 49–50, 59, 70, 87, 89
Albert Einstein College of Medicine (AECOM), 17–18, 62–63
Alcoholism. *See* Substance abuse services
Ambulatory care. *See also* Clinics; Community health care centers; Primary care
  emergency room (ER), 13, 15, 16, 35, 41, 52, 84, 95
  and international medical graduates (IMGs), 2, 16
  Lutheran Hospital, 71
  Medicaid Mills, *16t*, 42, 92–93
  outpatient department (OPD), 16, 41, 84
  provision by AHCs, 126
  public/private providers, 2, 15–22, 37–42
Ambulatory Care Network Corporation (ACNC)
  and Medicaid, 18, 67–68
  and nurse practitioners (NPs), 66, 67
  and primary care, 65–68
  Products of Ambulatory Care (PACs), 66
Ambulatory sensitive condition (ASC), 84, 114
Association of American Medical Colleges (AAMC), 2
Average annual per capita cost (AAPCC), 9, 63–64, 85, 94–95, 106–7
Axelrod, David, 5, 43, 59, 124–25

Martin Luther King, Jr. Center, 61
Medicaid. *See also* Medicaid managed
care; Medicare
and Ambulatory Care Network Corporation (ACNC), 18, 67–68
average annual per capita cost
(AAPCC), 63–64, 85, 94–95,
106–7
for blind/disabled, 50, 59, 60
characteristics of New York State
program, 1
and Columbia-Presbyterian Medical
Center, 17–18, 64–65
eligibility, 43
enrollment, 9–10, 12
general impact of, 3–4, 23
and Health and Hospitals Corporation (HHC), 19, 20, 37, 72–74,
104, 109–10, 122, 129
and health care quality, 6, 16, 47, 63
impact on elderly, 6, 48–49, 50–51,
53, 54, 59
impact on hospitals, 26–28, 38, 52,
55–57, 58–59
impact on physicians, 1, 54–55, 58,
89–91, 124
and Lutheran Hospital, 69–71, 86–
87
Medicaid Mills, *16t*, 42, 92–93
and Montefiore Medical Center, 63–
64
and nursing homes, 6, 22, 29, 51, 52,
53, 54, 59
and physicians
Medicaid managed care. *See also* Medicaid; Medicare
compulsory enrollment in, 87–88
funding of graduate medical education (GME), 100–101, 129
and health care destabilization, 105,
107–8, 118–19
and health care quality, 84–85
impact on health care employment,
100, 105
impact on hospitals, 97–100, 105
initial attempt at, 83–84
Medicaid Managed Care Act (1991),
17, 22, 84–87
patient orientation to, 95
physician participation in, 89–95

and primary care, 87–95
recruitment for, 95–96
for "special needs" population, 87,
89, 96–97
termination from, 96
voluntary enrollment in, 84–87, 95–
96
Medicaid Managed Care Act (1991),
17, 22, 84–87
Medicaid Mills, *16t*, 42, 92–93
and international medical graduates
(IMGs), 93
Medical Care Facilities Financing Authority (MCFFA), 44, 75–76
Medical education. *See* Academic health
centers (AHCs); Affiliation contracts; Graduate medical education
(GME); International medical graduates (IMGs); *specific schools*
Medically Underserved Areas (MUAs),
92
Medicare. *See also* Medicaid; Medicaid managed care
and biomedical research, 6
funding of graduate medical education (GME), 56, 62–63, 110–11
funding of international medical
graduates (IMGs), 2
and health care quality, 6, 16, 47,
63
impact on elderly, 3–4, 6, 29, 48–49,
50–51, 53, 59
impact on hospitals, 26–28, 38, 52,
55–57, 58–59
impact on physicians, 54–55, 58, 90
and Montefiore Medical Center, 63–
64
Mental health, 7, 69, 87, 96–97
Methadone Maintenance Treatment
Program (MMTP), 18
MetroPlus, 37, 83
Metropolitan Health Plan, 83
Metropolitan Health Plus, 74
Mitchell, Maria K., 109
Montefiore Medical Center
administrative management, 63–64
Bronx Health Plan (BHP), 17, 22,
63–64
community health care centers, 61–
62, 63–64, 68